Jutta Mattau

Tibetan
Power Yoga

The Essence of All Yogas
A Tibetan Exercise for Physical Vitality

LOTUS LIGHT
SHANGRI-LA

1st English Edition 1997
© by Lotus Light Publications
Box 325, Twin Lakes, WI 53181, USA
The Shangri-La Series is published in cooperation
with Schneelöwe Verlagsberatung, Federal Republic of Germany
© 1996 by Windpferd Verlagsgesellschaft mbH, Aitrang, Germany
Translated by Christine M. Grimm
Cover design by Kuhn Grafik, Digitales Design, Zurich
Interior illustrations: Ute Rossow
ISBN 0-914955-30-6
Library of Congress Catalog Number 97-71447

Printed in USA

Tibetan
Power Yoga

Table of Contents

Foreword

How good it is that there are people who open our eyes for the truly elementary things of this world.

My first prominent teachers were my parents, patient and loving as they were. In school, we naturally had a great many good and bad teachers. Although we studied more for the exams than for life at that time, these teachers were also—considered in retrospect—very important.

Later on, I used my own criteria to look for my own teachers. The spotlight of my attention often focused on eccentric people, who then became a type of model for me. I admired their personalities and tried to be like them.

These were people like the political refugee from South Africa. He had been a professor there, taught at a university, and came from a rich family. Because of his view of equality for the races he had to flee at that time. I got to know him as he made his rounds through the bars of our city with a bouquet of roses in his hand. I learned much about the transience of wealth from him, and he taught me the courage to speak.

A little cuddly bundle on four legs also became a friend and reminded me time and again of the unbridled delight of carefree happiness.

In India I later encountered ascetics, noble men with sparkling, lively eyes. They kindled their life's fire through disciplined meditation and renunciation of attachment to worldly luxury.

The beggar, who lived from alms and plucked Spanish flamenco on his guitar in the park of our city in the evening, also crossed my path. His only possessions were just a few plastic bags and his guitar.

And then there was naturally Uncle Ludwig, a victor in terms of business, from whom I was also permitted to learn.

Actually, I have had many teachers and role models for my life.

Like pearls on a chain, the experiences of a life are strung together. If some of the pearls were to be missing, then the chain would be incomplete. The overall picture couldn't be created in the same way as it appears today. Yet, there are some particularly beautiful gemstones strung onto the chain of every life. Even from the distance, they glitter conspicuously, and the chain would only be half as valuable without them.

This book is about one of these gemstones. Its story is about the Tibetan way of looking at life since the path of my life later led me to the highlands of Tibet. Today I can say that I found a key that opened the door to deeper spirituality for me in Tibet. There's no question that the path into the inner realms is long. However, once you have taken the first step on it, you will continue to follow the trail of perception. Many temptations wait on both sides of the path, inviting you to rest. In other places, there are dangers. Raging rivers tear us with them and perilous abysses open up. These cliffs can only be conquered with sharpened senses. But once this "red thread" has been taken up, it winds its way straight to the endless horizon.

Tsering Norbu led me on the path to my own personal red thread. This Buddhist monk taught me to follow an inner path without having to give up my previous life. Wisdom lies concealed in every soul and waits only to be revealed.

In addition to the many profound pieces of wisdom, Tsering Norbu shared a special yoga exercise with me. This yoga has been considered the essence of all secret and highest yogas for thousands of years. Even today, it is practiced by every common Tibetan citizen in the monastery, as well as by the monks in the lonely cave hermitages of the Himalayas.

People who practice this yoga on a regular basis can develop the perfect merging of mind, body, and soul. Tsering Norbu once said: "This exercise is the essence of all yogas in a bud. The perfect knowledge of Buddha is reflected within it."

Tsering Norbu called this yoga the "Tibetan Power Yoga", it is the "Tibetan Prostration", similar to a great, strong wave.

In addition to other treasures, the story of this book describes the art of this prostration. I have portrayed it here as I saw the Tibetan's practice it and as I have come to understand it through my own years of experiences with it.

From the Western perspective, "prostration" first sounds uncomfortable. We spontaneously think of subjugation, and we make such an effort to "be above it all." Who wants to be submissive or made to knuckle under?

Without a doubt: Self-assertion is not just useful but necessary in order to make it through life. The practice of prostration in no way violates this natural pride.

Yet, it's worthwhile to take a look at the word "prostration" without any reservations. In more exact terms, prostration is the radical form of a bow to something worth admiring. It shows respect for qualities that we would like to have ourselves. The term "prostration" is meant to, and should be, understood solely in this positive sense.

So please let go of the possibly unpleasant tinge that this term may have for you. Instead, open up to its actual meaning. Although it's true that the word "bow" would have sounded softer, I didn't use it because it is still too moderate. The person who practices this form of yoga actually lies stretched out completely on the ground—in full devotion to the harmonious unity of body, mind, and soul.

Open yourself up to this adventure!

Beginning of a Long Journey

Revolutionary events in life seldom announce themselves with kettle drums and trumpets. It's usually some little thing that starts an important matter rolling. You just have to be at the proper place at the appropriate moment and encounter the right person there. Everything else then happens practically on its own.

Who isn't familiar with these situations that suddenly change so many things? Often, the significance of such a moment only becomes clear much later, and a person even will remember these, initially small, incidents years later. Had they not been such an incisive turning point in life, they would have long been forgotten.

Such a moment that changed my life—and ultimately led to this book—was a telephone call from my friend Ingrid...

The phone rang piercingly. I hated being disrupted when I was at work, but I was expecting an important call. So I quickly pressed the "save" key on the computer, stumbled over a pile of books scattered on the floor to the phone, and picked up the receiver. It wasn't the caller I'd expected, but Ingrid.

"I thought you're not answering at all anymore," she greeted me impatiently. "Imagine, there's going to be a slide show about Tibet tonight. Want to come with me?"

"No time," was my mechanical response, "I have to deliver my manuscript in two days and still have a lot to do on it."

"You're really strange. The only time that something interesting takes place in this small town you chicken out," Ingrid grumbled. "So do what you want. I'm going in any case."

I hesitated for a moment. The Buddhist culture of Tibet had always fascinated me. I hardly missed a television report about the "Roof of the World," as Tibet is often described in picturesque terms. Besides, a small diversion from work would do me good.

"You win," I heard myself saying, "I'll come with you."

That evening, I took a colorful series of pictures with me into my dreams. Nomads with goats and herds of yaks that wandered through the endless deserts of stone. Somber monasteries in which monks mumbled unspoken wishes in endless prayers. The face of a Tibetan woman as she laughs refreshingly into the camera. The faithful who throw themselves onto the ground in front of a temple time and again. That night, I took my first long trip through the highlands of Tibet.

Days passed, the manuscript had long been completed, and I now turned to the next assignment. But I somehow didn't have the right momentum. Something important was rumbling inside my feelings. But what should it be? With increasing frequency, I caught myself thinking of the pictures I had drank in on the evening of the slide show. There was a growing longing inside me for Tibet. But the earliest possible time for the next vacation was in six months. And anyway, I had wanted to go to Spain this time. Even a trip to Asia, which I sometimes liked to take, was no longer of interest to me. I had planned a time of total recuperation after the recent period of stress resulting from my work. I just wanted to do nothing at all for once, what bliss!

Yet, during this night I dreamed that I bought an airplane ticket to Tibet. That was irritating. I deliberately ignored this hint from the subconscious as well and acted like nothing had happened. I was ultimately sensible enough to plan my life for myself! But the same dream kept repeating itself the following nights.

Then came that Tuesday morning. I sat in front of my cup of coffee, and the certainty suddenly penetrated me like a flash of lightning. Without a further thought, I ran to the telephone and called a travel agency. Five minutes later, a flight to Lhasa was booked in my name. And not in six months, but in three weeks.

"You did *what?*" Ingrid was aghast as I casually held the booking voucher under her nose that same evening. A moment later, she was grinning again.

"I actually thought I knew you well enough, but something like this..."

"That's what I thought about myself up to now. But believe me: I simply have to do it," I responded in a relaxed tone.

My life had actually taken what people call "an ordinary course" up to that time. I had a happy personal life, a lovable partner, good friends, and a profession that I found to be fulfilling. As a freelance journalist, I enjoyed more freedom than most other people. What more can you desire for yourself?

Yet, there was a great yearning deep inside of me, a longing to comprehend the mystery of life and the soul. It couldn't be put into words. Sometimes I felt the satisfaction in my life to be very much limited to superficial values. For example, what would happen when this nicely crafted scene, the friends, the partner, the job, one day collapsed? I didn't even risk thinking about it. In any case, I would be left standing there with empty hands.

It was clear to me that there must be a deeper meaning at the bottom of this facade of everyday life. This is why I liked to travel to foreign countries and become familiar with the philosophies of other cultures. I wanted to know what values and standards in life were important to other people. An unspoken yearning had long gotten a hold on me.

The following three weeks passed quickly. Thousands of little things still had to be taken care of. The biggest problem was placating my clients with their attitude of "how can you do this, and now of all times!"

To be quite honest about it, I couldn't permit myself this trip at all in terms of time. Annoyed voices hissed through the telephone receiver. Never before had they experienced me as being so unreliable. I had agreed to work for two or three magazines, and now the responsible editors had to look for someone else.

My friends and my partner were also irritated. "Why do you suddenly want to go to Tibet? Didn't you want to go to Spain?"

These were naturally the same questions that I also asked myself. Yet, when I was in bed at night and stared holes into the darkness, something strange happened: the holes turned into magical circles into which the pictures of Tibet zoomed. There were always the same colorful visions of the mountains, monasteries, and the solitude. No matter what power it was that had so completely surprised me here, my decision was the right one. I clearly felt it.

I had no idea of how to plan this four-week trip. Using a travel guide, I halfheartedly put together routes to the interesting places to see—and then dismissed the idea. I didn't even know myself what I was actually looking for there. I finally decided not to work out any route at all. I wanted to let myself "go with the flow" and be surprised.

As I got on the train to the airport, I finally looked at my coming adventure with the necessary dose of composure.

The first step into unknown Tibet had begun. Lhasa, a Chinese garrison city with a bustling atmosphere I wasn't enthusiastic about, had little to do with the Tibet that I was searching for. I didn't want to stay there any longer than I had to.

For this reason, I was particularly happy to talk to some Western tourists at the hotel bar one evening. Daniel, an Australian, was familiar with the area from earlier trips.

"Why don't you go to the mountain Kailash," Daniel suggested. "Kailash is one of the holiest places in the world. This mountain is the seat of the gods. The four mightiest rivers of Asia have their source there. Can you imagine the power this mountain emanates? Buddhists and Hindus dream of going on a pilgrimage there at least once in their lives. If you are looking for a spiritual place, then go to Kailash!"

The thought enticed me. Daniel described the travel route in detail for me that evening.

"But the trip is no picnic," he warned. "You'll need several days to get there. You can travel the first part of the journey with the public bus. For the remaining stretch, you must rent a jeep or, if that doesn't work, ride along on a truck."

"That doesn't matter. I have all the time in the world. And now I'm going to treat you to a beer."

The next morning, even before the first crow of the rooster, I was ready to take off. Namgyal, a friendly Tibetan with a weather-beaten face who worked at the hotel, accompanied me to the bus station. Because of the biting cold that was still in the air at this hour, he wore a long red wool coat and a fur cap on his head. "So, here we are. Have a good trip," said Namgyal, as we stood in front of the old rusty bus that I was supposed to get into. As he left, I cheerfully put my backpack on the roof and sat down in a window seat—an absolute privilege, as I later discovered. Shortly before the rattletrap jerked out of the bus station, it was chock—full and the passengers stood crammed tightly into the center aisle.

Leaning back relaxed in the seat, I let the highland's monotonous deserts of stone flow past me during the next few days. Here and there was a lonely village and traveling nomads on the road. The adventure of Tibet could now begin.

This day in the bus was the beginning of a long journey: a trip to Kailash, I thought at the time. I certainly didn't know that I wouldn't encounter the holy mountain during this tour. My excursion ended as quickly as it had begun, and just a few days later. I stayed until the end of my trip in this little city where the rattletrap bus spit me out after an unending ride. It wasn't for four weeks, as I had planned, but for an entire four months! This is where a new part of my journey began. The journey through inner worlds.

This town in Tibet really exists. However, it's name is unimportant because no one should come looking for this city.

The following story also exists in reality. I will tell it like it took place, and could have taken place. In a kaleidoscope of worlds, the visions merge with realities, and dreams and wide, awakeness shake hands.

Surprising Encounter

Never in life will I forget my first visit to this Tibetan monastery. After a good night's sleep following the long journey on the previous day, I entered the cold, dark room that morning. The tart smell of frankincense went up my nose even before I could see anything. I only perceived the silhouette of a monk in a corner of the room. He sat on a pillow on the ground, oblivious to the world. He mumbled mystic phrases in a monotonous sing-song voice while he evenly beat on a large drum. I paused for a moment and let the muffled sound echo within me.

When my eyes had become accustomed to the darkness, I recognized some statues representing deities on a table. What a great difference in the expressions on their faces! Some looked so friendly that I spontaneously had to laugh, and others made me shrink back in fear with their fearsome grimaces. One angry figure magically attracted me: her wide-open black eyes glowed with power, and she wore a chain of skulls around her neck. A red-yellow sea of flames blazed around the entire figure. Under her right foot, she energetically squashed a spindly creature. Was this the victory of good over evil, or the other way around? With relief I now recognized a familiar figure: a golden Buddha in the lotus position. Deeply immersed in thought, he held a beggar's dish in his hands. Buddha, a symbol for the essence of the perfect human spirit since the beginning of all time.

These figures played their teasing game with the observer, causing the strings of secret feelings to vibrate. The deeper I walked into the dark room, the more bewildering the world of my own gods and demons was as it unfolded inside of me. As if by a magician's hand, a beam of light suddenly fell through the mat window pane onto a golden, delicate figure: a women with opulent breasts, her body ornamented with turquoise, corals, and other glittering precious stones in a complete fusion of feminine suppleness. Equanimity and kindness emanated from her physical posture. Spellbound, I remained standing in front of this noble manifestation shining in pure gold at this moment, until the beam of light broke and she sank back into the twilight.

I had visited many temples during the past seven years on my trips to Asia—temples of Hindus in India and Buddhist monasteries in Japan and China. All of them were interesting, but this room here touched something deep within my soul.

I suddenly felt unwell between all the colorful figures, the significance of which was so mysterious and simultaneously so familiar to me. Confused, I took another look around this mysterious place and then purposefully walked out to the monastery courtyard.

But what a trick my fantasy now played on me again: before my eyes was exactly the same picture that I had seen just four weeks ago in the slide show. I blinked a bit, but the picture remained. This time, it was reality. In the pale morning light, with their faces always turned to the monastery, women and men threw the entire length of their bodies to the ground and got back up, only to sink to the ground once again. At the same time, they incessantly murmured secretive verses.

I sat down on the cold stone steps and pondered on how abruptly dreams sometimes come true. Soon I was able to direct my attention to the scene. I noticed that some of the older Tibetans practiced this flow of movement with an ease that revealed unbelievable physical fitness. At that moment, I couldn't think of any older person at home that I believed capable of a similar feat. Did these people keep themselves so flexible with these prostrations? It was a very interesting question. I was starting to get cold and returned to my boardinghouse in a contemplative mood.

The house was located a bit outside the lively downtown area. I especially loved the view from my window of the large white shrine. The massive foundational walls of this Buddhist shrine tapered increasingly upwards. Its filigreed, light-red tip ended in a metallic umbrella, the small brass plates of which chimed delicately in the wind. It made the loveliest sound when a fresh breeze from the city drifted up into the mountains in the evening. The gigantic willow tree in front of this shrine could probably have told a long story of its life. Its trunk had become rotten with age, and the broken-off branches had left deep wounds. Now it leaned in fatigue against a massive stone wall. While this worn-down giant wistfully reminded me of the transience of all being, the solid cut stone of the shrine apparently wanted to defy this principle. It constantly shone in fresh white because the neighbors painted it every year. An owl had built its nest in the branches of the old willow. Sending its lonely cry up to the heavens, it rocked me to sleep at night as I rested in my bed. Then, the excited sparrows that were permitted to occupy the tree during the day chirped in the morning. These were melancholy harmonies between the cycle of growth and decay, a balm for the soul.

In the afternoon I ambled through the market square, wanting to drink in some impressions of this city since I had planned to continue on to Kailash the next morning. On the streets I recognized some of the people I had seen in front of the temple that morning. I looked into their clear, open eyes. These eyes reflected happy and powerful souls. Wasn't it amazing that precisely the Tibetans had such cheerfulness within them? The political situation of the country was difficult enough: the occupation of their nation by the Chinese had brought the people here into deeply humiliating and often desperate situations. Politically uncomfortable people disappeared into prisons, and the suspicion towards the Chinese soldiers present everywhere was also very clearly perceptible in this city.

Despite all this, these people appear to be masters of the art of living. I presume that the art of being able to love life despite all the adverse circumstances was related to their deep Buddhist faith. Perhaps the prostrations in front of the temple were also somehow related to this feeling of life. I vaguely sensed that these exercises were much more than just physical fitness. But what role did they play?

While I strolled through the city without any objective, I became certain of this much: from now on I would no longer be "just" a tourist. I was on the track of a very personal secret, the mystery of which I wanted to solve. My dreams had been correct after all. I couldn't depart from this temple where I had seen the prostrations for the first time this morning.

Now the mountain Kailash was no longer important. I spontaneously decided to remain in this city. Relieved, I ran back to my boardinghouse in order to tell the woman who owned it that I would stay longer in my room.

During the following days, I explored the cozy little town in which I had ended up. Although it had no particular sights of interest, the atmosphere was friendly and soon felt good to me. I naturally spent several hours every day at the temple.

One morning, an older monk spoke to me there. I had already seen him often as I sat on the stone steps and watched the faithful Tibetans at their prostrations. This man came shortly after six every morning and made a pilgrimage of several rounds around the temple, attentively turning the countless prayer wheels that were built like pearls into the wall around the building. Afterwards, he left. He never appeared to notice me.

Yet, on this morning the monk headed directly for me. To my astonishment, he spoke English quite well: "You have been here often. Tourists usually do not stay that long in this city." He made himself comfortable next to me on the stone steps. "Why are you here?"

How could I explain it? Yet, the words already poured out of me at the same moment: I told him of my longing for Tibet that I had had since I saw the slide show. I described the deep peace evoked within me by the atmosphere of this temple.

I spoke of the longing in my soul and the heartfelt wish of capturing a glimpse of this secret.

With patience, the monk listened attentively to my torrent of words until I abruptly paused. For a moment, I was ashamed that I had told a stranger so much. He had opened a tap for all these things that were so important to me. When I finished speaking, there was a moment of silence between us.

Then the monk said: "Visit me this afternoon around three o'clock. I will initiate you into the prostrations."

He introduced himself as Tsering Norbu and wrote his address on a piece of paper for me.

"Until then, stranger," he curtly finished our conversation.

Even before I could say something in response, he had hurried down the stairs and disappeared. I could hardly know at that time that Tsering Norbu would not only teach me the essence of life for the next three weeks, but for many years.

I excitedly waited for the afternoon, but the time slipped by too slowly that day. Finally, it was time for me to take the path to his house in the old part of town. Tsering Norbu already waited at the door of his house and waved to me like an old acquaintance. He asked me to enter.

The room in which the monk lived was a small, spartanically furnished chamber. The furnishings consisted of three chairs, a bed, and a closet. In one corner, which Tsering Norbu called his "kitchen," was a gas cooker.

As the Tibetan tradition required, he first boiled a pot of buttered tea before we sat down. Tsering Norbu started a casual conversation, which quickly made my nervousness vanish. During the course of this conversation, he revealed to me that he had lived in America for seven years—which is why he spoke English so well!

"But why America?" I wondered.

"That's a long story, " responded the monk, "but I will tell it to you in brief. As you certainly know, thousands of Tibetans fled to foreign countries after the Chinese invasion of Lhasa in the year 1959. Above all, they went to India and Nepal. I was also one of these, and I first settled in Nepal. Even at that time, the first Lamas traveled to the West in order to teach Tibetan Buddhism there. The first Buddhist centers were also established at that time. I believe this was a good thing. The people in the West are very hungry for old, deep wisdom."

Tsering Norbu took a noisy sip of his oily buttered tea.

"An old friend, who was also a Lama, wrote me at that time from America. He asked me to come and give lectures on Buddhism at one of these centers. Yes, I learned a great deal at that time. It's astonishing how many differences there are between life in America and life in Tibet. Yet, whether in America or Tibet, people everywhere are driven by the same fears, desires, and hopes. Yes, the feelings are truly the same in all people, no matter where they live on the Earth. They simply express themselves in different ways.

Well, at some point I had a longing for my homeland. I believe that the same thing happens to every person when he gradually grows old and wants to return to his roots. That's why I decided to return to Tibet at that time."

Tsering Norbu suddenly interrupted his story: "I know that you are practically bursting with impatience, so we now want to talk about the prostrations. First, the most important thing: the prostration is the key with which you can find your inner and outer equilibrium. Just as in a bud, all essential yoga exercises are concentrated within it. This is why it is perfect!

His words flowed into me like honey. I heaved a sign of relief. When this wise man spoke in this manner, then it must also be true. The prostrations could bring me to the path that I had searched for so long. My intuition on that first morning in front of the temple hadn't deceived me.

While I dwelled on this delight, the monk vigorously got up from his chair to get some cookies. The strength of his body and youthful smoothness of his movements caught my eye. Up to that time, I had only seen such a "round" sense of physical expression in a few young men. At the same time, his face, wrinkled and weather-beaten from the raw climate, revealed the maturity of his years. How old could Tsering Norbu be?

"My age?" he laughed. "You modern people always need numbers to hold onto. But, alright: I'm 75 years old or even older. I don't know my exact age. But I have practiced the prostrations every day since my youth—even in America. I have kept my body fit and my mind flexible with them."

This was becoming even more fascinating for me!

"I'm burning to learn more about this wonderful yoga exercise," I exclaimed curiously.

Tsering Norbu strictly refused: "You cannot understand everything yet. Your habits of thought still stand in your way."

"That's not true! I'm completely receptive," I contradicted. "And anyway: I have to go home in three weeks. By then I want to know what these prostrations are all about. After all, I also want to practice the exercises at home."

But with this point I thoroughly got nowhere with the old Tibetan.

"Ah, you are really an offspring of the West. You always want to know everything right away. You are all too much controlled by your minds and believe that you can comprehend everything with your intelligence. But that's not how it works. I will naturally give you the tools to take along with you and explain the prostrations and their philosophy to you. But you can truly understand the exercise only with your heart.

This is why I seriously ask you to take your time and learn to comprehend with your intuition and your heart. Only when you can understand from the depths of your soul will the practice of prostration change you. However, I promise you this: It's worth it."

With these words, Tsering Norbu went back to the "kitchen" and put on another pot of water for the tea. Now the silence felt good. Relaxed, I leaned back in the chair and noticed for the first time the cosy atmosphere that this simple room emanated. In the meanwhile, my teacher briefly left the room and brought a red flower with him, which he laid on the table in front of me without a comment, but with a sly wink of the eye.

After refilling our bowls with the steaming buttered tea, he sat down and picked up his story once again.

"I want to give you an example of this that my students in the West always understood quite well: Take this flower in your hand and look at it. At first, you can see what color it has, how many petals and blossoms are on it, and, if you are knowledgeable about botany, you will even know its Latin name. This is intellectual comprehension. But looking at this flower with the heart means you sit down in front of it for a long time and mentally put yourself into this flower. At some point, you will understand this little, inconspicuous flower in another way, comprehend its transience, grasp it in its sense of being a flower.

From that moment on, this flower is unique for you, and you will remember it for a long time to come. This is exactly the same with all other things that you encounter. It always depends on your inner, deep motivation with which you carry something out. And this is exactly how it is with the prostrations. On the one hand, they are an outstanding physical exercise. However, you will only discover its unique depth when you have looked at it and felt it for a longer time.

So, now our flower first needs some water so that it does not die of thirst."

He had caught me. I actually had hoped to receive some sort of directions for use that I could follow.

As if he had guessed my thoughts, Tsering Norbu continued: "I will make you an offer. I will always teach you just as much as you can comprehend at one time. And furthermore," he added with a smile, "I know precisely that you will come back to Tibet time and again in order to learn more. Yet, what I said before is the most important lesson for you at the moment: Always be present in your heart and have patience with yourself."

My lesson was over for today. Tsering Norbu got up, smoothed his red robe, and said good-bye to me with the promise: "Tomorrow we will start with the first lesson on the prostrations."

Now I was outside again, and the twilight slowly set in. The fresh air did me good. I pensively wandered through the narrow lanes, observing children at play and watching the dealers pack their goods. As Tsering Norbu had suggested, I tried to see with more than just my eyes. I wanted to let the mood have its effect and flow into my belly. My ears listened carefully and heard the dogs bark and the people chat. My nostrils opened up and drew in the musty-sweetish smell of the alleys. The tips of my fingers became tender and felt the raw plaster of the house wall as I walked along it.

Inspired by all the exciting stimuli, I let myself be enticed into a small cookshop by a spicy cloud of fragrance. I was ravenous. In a great mood, I ordered a big portion of my favorite Tibetan dish: fried noodles and vegetables.

Softness of the Wave

The next morning I met Tsering Norbu again at the temple. However, he just briefly waved to me from the distance. I observed the way he concentrated on turning one prayer wheel after the other on his rounds. Now I knew that scrolls with Buddhist texts were inside these cylinders. When a person starts them turning, they begin to emanate their positive power and pass it on to the believers. Buddhists even say that the energy of these texts increases one-thousand fold when the wheels are set into motion.

On his way back to the exit of the temple courtyard, my friend briefly walked by me: "Come this afternoon again at the same time. I will be expecting you." He seemed to still be immersed in meditation and was apparently not in the mood for a chat.

When I arrived at his place at 3 o'clock, there was already a pot of steaming buttered tea on the table, next to a water glass with the red flower. Tsering Norbu was more serious today than he was yesterday. As soon as I had sat down on my chair he came to the point:

"For the prostration there is an inner and an outer path," he lectured. Then he pointed to the flower.

"Remember what I said yesterday. In accordance with this, the outer path is the physical exercise itself. The inner path is portrayed by the thoughts and feelings that you develop during the exercise. Both parts are inseparably connected with each other. Since we are starting slowly, I will now explain the outer path to you."

In order to make room, Tsering Norbu cleared away the table and pushed both of our chairs into the corner. "You have observed the essence of all yogas often enough in front of the temple. It is very simple. Come, the best thing is for you to practice yourself right away."

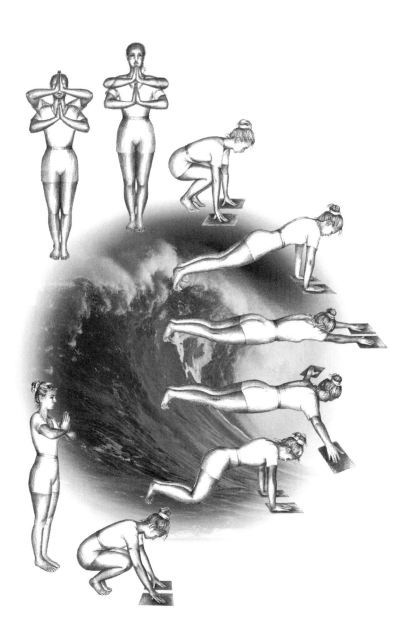

With a quickly beating heart, I stood on the free surface and looked at the monk expectantly.

"Stand there as straight as a candle and place the palms of your hands together in front of your chest. This is the starting position in which you first collect yourself. Now lift your hands up to the top of your head. In a flowing motion, bring them back down over your throat to your chest. The top of the head, throat, and chest are chakra points. Pause briefly at each of them. Yes, that's good. Now open your hands and bend down with slightly bent knees in the direction of the ground. Move forwards on the palms of your hands until you are stretched out at full length on the ground."

In the meantime, the monk had placed two pieces of cloth on the ground at both sides of my body so I could put my hands on them. With this cloth, I could smoothly glide forwards. So now I was laying fully stretched out on the floor.

"Now," I heard his voice, "don't remain in this position. Move your arms, stretched out and in a wide circular arc, back to your hips. Then get up immediately: first on your knees, then squatting, and then stand up in a completely erect position. Now return to the starting position by placing your hands together in front of your chest. See, that was it. It isn't difficult at all, is it?"

I beamed at him. I was secretly even a bit proud, but I was careful not to say this to Tsering Norbu. With his instructions, I was permitted to repeat the exercise two more times.

"Be sure that your feet are always on the same spot," the monk admonished me. In my eagerness, I had actually slid a good stretch backwards.

"And something else: be sure that your stomach doesn't touch the floor too soon. It should only rest on it when your hands are almost stretched out all the way. And don't cheat yourself by first getting on your knees and then flowing forwards. This would cut the power of this exercise in half."

We pushed the furniture back into place and sat down.

"Do I have to pay attention to my breathing?" I asked.

I knew that breathing is very important in Indian yoga exercises. He said it wasn't important here.

"We Tibetans don't pay attention to the breathing rhythm in this exercise. But I think that it would help you at the start. When you support them with your breathing, the individual motions become more conscious. Come, it's best for you to try it out right away." We once again pushed the furniture to the side of the room.

Once again, I stood with my feet next to each other and placed my hands together in front of my chest. Tsering Norbu lectured: "Before you begin the cycle, take two conscious breaths. When exhaling, very powerfully expel the air from your lungs. Imagine that you are ejecting the tensions of body and mind in the form of black air. The actual exercise only begins after this fundamental cleansing.

Each prostration includes inhaling twice and exhaling twice. Gently inhale as you stand and touch the top of your head, mouth, and heart with your folded hands. While doing this, imagine that the radiant energy of the cosmos is flowing into your body. Slowly exhale while gliding down to the floor. While you move your arms in the shape of an arc to your hips and stand up, inhale once again. And finally: when you are standing, exhale once again.

When exhaling, imagine that all the tensions are streaming out of your body. At the same time, negative thoughts and feelings are also flowing away."

I was now somewhat out of breath and asked Tsering Norbu for a glass of water.

"Did you feel how the prostration depicts the movement of a wave?" he wanted to know. I shook my head. After all, I had been too busy with the details.

"In the future, try to feel your body to be a wave during the exercise, as a soft, flowing movement."

My teacher decided it was now time for a break. A good idea! I wanted to get some fresh air and strolled back and forth in front of the house for a few minutes. The narrow streets were practically empty of all life. Just a few dogs dozed in the mild sun of the late afternoon. Tsering Norbu was already waiting for me when I came back into the house.

"You should get to know an interesting effect of the prostrations. They cleanse the energy channels in the body. The impulses of the autonomous nervous system begin to flow evenly so that the system can regenerate throughout the entire organism."

The monk paused for a moment, then added: "And the essence of all yogas has one more unbelievable effect: you will strengthen your body with the prostrations. Look at me. I am living proof. But I warn you: your muscles will hurt at the beginning. Start slowly and do not overstrain yourself. This is not at all a matter of achieving the best performance. You would probably achieve the opposite with this attitude."

"How many prostrations are recommended?" I wanted to know.

"At the beginning, fifteen are completely adequate. But do these carefully. Now it's important that your body learns to move properly. Observe how you depict a wave-shaped flow. Later, when the movement has turned into second nature for you, you will also be mentally involved. But the time is not ripe for this. Here is your first assignment: go to the temple tomorrow morning and do this exercise just like you learned it today."

My heart slid down to my knees. I was actually supposed to practice my first prostrations while subject to the curious glances of the Tibetans? I would give myself away. Tsering Norbu calmed me down: "Have trust and open yourself for what will happen. Fear is only the feeling of insecurity about situations with which you are not familiar."

As if *that* should be a comfort to me. However, after I mentally measured my little hotel room and had to admit that there wasn't enough room in it to learn the exercise in privacy, I yielded to his instructions.

"All right, I'll do it. See you tomorrow, Tsering Norbu."

I walked to the temple. As I had hoped, there were actually some people there practicing the prostrations. I sat down on the stone steps and watched them. I imagined myself standing among them and feeling good. My fear usually disappears when I let a difficult impending situation take form in front of my inner eye and decide that everything will work out well. This is positive visualization. I gradually calmed down. However, it occurred to me that all the Tibetans used pieces of cloth in order to slide forwards on the smooth stone floor. I still had to organize these for my dress rehearsal the next morning.

Back at the boardinghouse, I asked the owner for her help.

"No problem," she laughed. "You simply take two pieces of sturdy cotton or linen material. The cloth should be thick enough, at best sewn double and padded. If not, the palms of your hands will quickly become unpleasantly hot when you slide forwards repeatedly. For beginners in particular, and especially those who have delicate hands like you do, sliding forwards on cloth works the best."

She opened a closet and got out two pieces of material. "These are mine. You can use them for the time being."

"Thank you very much, that's very nice of you. But I'd like to get my own right away," I responded.

One hour later I bought two lovely wine-red pieces of linen, folded in half and well-padded, for a few cents at the cloth store in the old part of town.

That evening, while I wrote a letter to my friend Ingrid, the landlady knocked on the door of my room. She held a blanket under her arm.

"Here, take this blanket to the temple tomorrow. Fold it so that it's narrow and put it on the ground in front of you. This will better pad your body, particularly the knees, against the wooden floor. When you have done many prostrations, you will see that it's too hard without a blanket." The woman was really quite friendly.

The next morning, I started off for the temple in the pale light of the dawn. I was rather excited. Since I wanted to attract as little attention as possible, I retreated to the furthest corner of the place. I hoped to remain unobserved there. My lovely vision of the day before, standing between all the others with composure, unfortunately evidenced little power at the moment. Darn, the salesman from the cloth shop was already on his way over to me. I hadn't noticed that he was also practicing his prostrations a few steps away from me.

"Nice to see you here," he grinned curiously. I nodded to him, but hurried to add: "I tried it yesterday for the first time."

"If you want, I'll help you a bit. We can stand next to each other and do the exercise together. What do you think?" I accepted his help in getting started with relief.

"Let's go a bit further toward the front," he suggested. "You don't need to hide in the corner here."

We found a free spot between other people who were practicing. I carefully placed the blanket about 30 centimeters in front of my feet. I put both pieces of cloth to the left and right of it. Now things could get started.

I stood in the erect beginning position, as Tsering Norbu had explained it to me. I slowly folded my hands and raised them up to my forehead, concentrating on my breathing. Then I brought my hands down to my mouth and then to my heart. I opened my eyes in order to find the pieces of cloth. I quickly stole a glance at the cloth salesman. He stood next to me and observed me attentively. In a flowing movement, I now brought my palms in front of me. My stomach muscles were completely tensed now. It reminded me of the exertion in doing push-ups, with the stomach and arm muscles carrying the weight of the entire body. I gently let my body glide into a stretched-out position on the ground.

"Don't remain on the floor," said Tsering Norbu's voice

inside my head. "Bring the hands to the hips in a wide circular arc and then stand up."

I did two more prostrations. I had the feeling of carrying out the exercise in the right way. My neighbor also praised me: "You do that well. However, you shouldn't make a pause in the motion between the individual prostrations. Let them merge with each other in a soft flow." He then departed with: "We'll see each other again."

I was thankful for the man: He gave me the certainty that I could do the exercise properly even without Tsering Norbu's help.

But this just couldn't be true! Even before the tenth prostration I was out of breath. My heart began to beat fast and a heat wave shot into my head. How did the others manage this exertion with such ease? Most of all, how do the older people do it? Hats off to them, I still had much to learn. A fit of ambition came over me since I was still young and actually fit: So I did about 25 more prostrations before I finally rolled up the blanket while breathing heavily and then sat down on the steps. Fortunately, Tsering Norbu didn't see me in this state! At least I had gotten through my dress rehearsal in a half-way elegant manner.

Relieved, but still somewhat exhausted, I returned to the boardinghouse. The landlady came out of the kitchen as I rummaged around in my jacket pocket to find the key to my room. My satisfied glow revealed what she wanted to know.

"You shouldn't take a cold shower now," she advised. "If you cool down too quickly inside, the prostrations won't develop their full power in your body. A lukewarm shower would be fine. But the best thing to do is rub down your body with just a warm, damp towel and then wipe it with a dry towel afterwards.

I decided on the second-best possibility. Afterwards, I felt like a new woman. I was burning to tell Tsering Norbu about my experience. But the anticipated pleasure was premature since it already started in the early afternoon: a quiet ache first in the belly, then crawling up into my upper arms. The prophesied sore muscles were on their way!

Tsering Norbu just had a mocking grin for my suffering.

"Didn't I tell you that fifteen are enough at the start? You naturally had to overdo it again."

"But I enjoyed it so much. How should I have stopped?" I contradicted wearily.

"What good is it to you when your body is not prepared? Strictly limit yourself to fifteen exercises for the time being," he commanded. He got no argument from me.

"Since we are on the topic of overzealousness, a very typical problem of the West comes to mind for me," Tsering Norbu continued in a reconciliatory tone. It was clear that he wasn't really annoyed with me. He was more like a worried father who wants to protect his child from harm. We once again sat in his chamber, where I now felt completely at home.

"You know," the monk began, "I do not wish to hold a speech against ambition. Ambition is even a positive virtue so that people can fully utilize their abilities and rub against their boundaries. But, and this is my criticism, why does healthy ambition always have to turn into overexertion for you people in the West? You exceed the boundary of a healthy ability to perform by doing so."

I was impressed by the way that this old man put his finger on weak points with incisive attentiveness and simultaneously linked them with the ancient Tibetan wisdom.

Tsering Norbu appeared to be thinking for a moment before he continued to speak: "This ambition is related to a lack of patience. You have now lived for thirty-five years without once having done a prostration. But for us Tibetans it becomes second nature from early childhood on. Do you see the difference? How much do you actually expect of yourself! Always realistically recognize the point where you are right now. The path has always been there, and it will also always be there, so you can walk it with composure. There is no real reason to hurry.

But you people? You always want to have everything—and preferably right away. If something does not work out, your patience is soon exhausted. What appeared important to you a moment ago is now quickly thrown away. Much too quickly! And your plans had no opportunity to ripen in peace."

I listened in dismay. At the same time, a German saying occurred to me: "A thing well done can't be done quickly."

The older generation appears to have comprehended this wisdom of patience. But for our fast-moving generation it appears to have gradually been forgotten.

"How does this lack of patience come about?" I wanted to know from Tsering Norbu. It was fascinating how our conversations sometimes digressed from the original topic, the prostrations. However, when considered more closely, these were also a part of the spiritual exercises in which all the different aspects flowed together.

"Your impatience? It comes from a lack of self-love," the monk responded laconically. At the same time, he looked at me sharply from the corner of his eye. He was apparently waiting for my protest, which naturally came right away: "But that's not possible! Everyone tries, particularly in our society, to get the best for himself. That's precisely our problem: everyone is fighting for his own advantage. I would even speak of egotistic self-love."

Tsering Norbu thoroughly rejected the idea: "You may be right at the first glance. But once again, your eyes only perceive what is on the surface. Go one step further: does this, what you call "egotistic striving," make people happy? Think of all the heart attacks, cancers, allergies, and the many highly paid therapists and psychiatrists.

Suffering everywhere! Why can't so many people find their own happiness? I will tell you: because they don't like themselves. In the West, I constantly heard sentences like: 'I must fulfill these demands or expectations,' 'I should definitely take care of this today,' and so forth. So much 'should' and 'must'!"

A person who likes himself does not voluntarily subject himself to so much miserable pressure. The stress will become so immense at some point that all these duties can only be fulfilled with sharp elbows and broad shoulders. That hardly has anything to do with self-love. Do you understand what I mean?"

The monk paused for a moment. I suddenly had to laugh: I imagined that one of these sentences, spoken in complete seriousness, came from Tsering Norbu's lips. It was a grotesque caricature. He was so far removed from these types of demands on oneself. On the other hand, I knew enough people at home from whom such sentences sounded completely normal. Unfortunately, I could even hear my own voice among them.

"A person who constantly runs at full pressure and continuously places demands on himself will never be happy," the monk continued. "Tell your friends that they should learn to love themselves. Tell them that every human being is lovable. Even if he doesn't fulfill the demands that others place on him."

Every person should treat himself like his own child, in a loving and friendly way."

"Why should an adult treat himself like a child?" I was on the verge of not understanding anything anymore.

"Because the so-called rational mind is like a small child: it needs a long time in order to truly understand something. You can tell it today: 'I am a lovable person just as I am.' Then it will snarl back: 'But not as long as I have this flaw or that flaw.' Tell it: 'I am permitted to enjoy life.' Then it counters: 'But only when I have completed this work or been successful at that task.' Believe me: you are already worthy of love at this moment and are permitted to be happy without any ifs or buts. I know it may take years to truly understand this. But you will gradually develop more patience with yourself. This is why the rational mind is like a small child. It needs a long time to truly understand. Would you scold a child because it does not learn to walk in one day?" I shook my head. "Precisely. We practice with it until it can walk at some point. So always reprimand your inner child in a friendly manner. It will become easier each time. At some point you will be able to accept and love yourself as you are, no matter where you stand at the moment."

We continued to chat for a while, and then Tsering Norbu came back to the topic of the prostrations.

"Stay with fifteen exercises a day for the time being. After a week, you can increase them as you like. When you have adjusted to about forty prostrations, you will achieve a good physical and mental effect." Then he added with a grin: "Your sore muscles will hopefully curb your ambition a bit."

He had seen through me! In order to divert from the topic, I got up and walked back and forth a few steps in the room. The pain now reached down into my legs. My frustration just seemed to prod my friend's aggression.

"One more thing on the topic of ambition," he ruminated with a wry glance at the pitiful figure I made. "What I will now tell you should be a new challenge for your patience: the effect of the prostrations is namely all the greater the more of them you do.

In our tradition, almost every Tibetan does 100,000 prostrations at one time in his life. The right time for this is usually established by his spiritual teacher. Some fast during this intensive meditation or retreat into solitude."

His words were just beginning to flow quite well. However, after he took a look at my unhappy face he compassionately cut himself short. "Oh, dear. You've just come from twenty-five prostrations with a decent set of sore muscles to me, and I have to tell you such things. Well, first continue to be concerned with what you have been doing. Perhaps later the point in time will come when you have a desire to do the

100,000 prostrations. I only told you this to give you an idea of what extremes there are in the range of possibilities. This intensive practice strengthens the body and cleanses the spirit more than any other method. But as I said: you do not have to achieve a top performance. With the help of this exercise, gently guide your mind and body into the more subtle spheres, what more can you hope for?

Just as I almost was outside, Tsering Norbu pulled me back into the room again. "One more bit of advice. If you become tired during the exercise, rest while you are standing. Do not recuperate while squatting or lying on the floor. And something else: do the prostrations conscientiously. If not, it is better to forget them completely."

I spent a wonderful, enjoyable time during these days. When I didn't happen to be in the temple or with Tsering Norbu, I often sat on the terrace of my boardinghouse, enjoyed the view of the snow-white shrine, and leisurely browsed through books. The conversations with the monk sometimes touched me so deeply that I stayed awake in bed at night. Sometimes I thought that Tsering Norbu, this little town, and Tibet were all just a dream. Just the owl in the willow tree connected me with reality at these moments.

One sentence that Tsering Norbu said burned into my mind in particular: understand with your heart. What a tremendous potential of deeper insight into life was contained in this idea! Imagine: the eyes, ears, mouth, and nose no longer limit themselves as organs for the purpose of seeing, hearing, tasting, and smelling. They could much more serve as tools to practically photograph feelings and let them sink into the middle of the heart.

At some moments I believed that I already comprehended this art of deep sensitivity: like a lightly passing breeze, fragile and intangible. Words would shatter this magic that embeds itself on such a fine level.

This is why Tsering Norbu still held back his thoughts about the deeper correlations of the prostrations: "You must learn to first understand the things on the coarse, then on the finer levels. Always go from the outside to the inside. First comprehend the process of the prostration," he had said. "Then you can penetrate more deeply into the mental, spiritual, and emotional aspects of it. I can only explain to you what happens in the mind theoretically. You will only truly comprehend it through regular practice." I was very curious about what exciting experiences were still waiting for me in Tibet.

I always walked to the temple every morning in a cheerful mood. The annoying soreness in my muscles had gone away after a few days and my condition had improved noticeably. I was long part of the permanent "team" of people who were there every day. The others always gave me a friendly nod. Unfortunately, we didn't talk much since everyone concentrated on his own exercises. Then that strange day came.

It happened two weeks after my arrival in Tibet: As always, I carefully spread out my blanket on this floor in front of me on this clear morning. The two little wine-red clothes were next to it on both sides. As always, I did the same ritual: hands above the face to the chest, gliding forwards on the ground, lying there completely stretched out, following the wide circular arc, and then getting up again. Then everything from the beginning again, very evenly and quickly.

Suddenly it was there: the great wave. It was a very round wave that flowed harmoniously. The mind merged with the body in this monotonous up-and-down motion. The outside world melted away into a blur of glittering, colorful dots. I had no idea how long this trance lasted. Darn, I forgot to count again! But that didn't matter anymore. I wanted to swim in this flowing feeling as long as possible.

It was only the fast beating of my heart that brought me back to reality; the colorful dots formed themselves back into people, trees, the temple, and the pavement stones. I ended the exercise for now. I didn't tell Tsering Norbu anything about "my wave." He certainly would have found my enthusiasm to be exaggerated since the prostration was a "simple wave movement" for him. The Tibetans think little of our Western emotionality, Tsering Norbu once mockingly called it sentimentalism, and the tendency to mystify everything that could possibly be mystified. They were just as reluctant to speak about their own emotions and feelings. I often couldn't understand them at all.

The Proud Mountain

Yet, in the course of the next days I ran into a problem for which I urgently needed Tsering Norbu's advice. I now felt very much at home in the wave movement. It was a familiar feeling of happiness that triggered a deep inner fulfillment. But then, in the middle of an exercise, I stopped short. A feeling of reluctance to have to throw myself onto the ground in the next moment arose within me.

I didn't want to throw myself into the dust! And in front of whom should I actually prostrate myself? I stubbornly remained standing in my starting position and observed the others uncomprehendingly as they harmoniously carried out their exercises—as if nothing had happened. Bits of thoughts about "subjugation" and "degradation" raced through my head. Totally grim, I worked myself into this mental confusion. I thought about my German friends. How astonished they would have been if they could have seen me in such a curious situation here: sweating in front of a Tibetan temple, lying on the ground every ten seconds. No, I certainly didn't need to throw myself into the dust.

I finally pulled myself together (German perfectionism sometimes really doesn't hurt) and completed the prostrations conscientiously, but tenaciously. For once, I was glad that I just had to do twenty exercises and could now roll up the blanket.

I angrily marched home and took a long shower. In order to divert myself, I fell into a shopping frenzy. In the old part of town, I found a vintage Tibetan teapot made of brass with endless good-luck knots hammered into it. In the same store I purchased two wooden bowls with lids in which tsampa, Tibetan barley flour, is stored. I wanted to put them as ornaments into my glass cabinet at home, where I keep various souvenirs from Asia. In case this "Tibet trip" got me completely stuck, I wanted to at least take along a few nice souvenirs of the journey.

I no longer know why I bought that green blouse in the clothing store: cheap synthetic fibers, imported from China, and I already regretted my acquisition as I unpacked the bag back in my room.

Had I possibly deluded myself into believing in the magic of the prostrations? Behind my angry facade, I felt dread in my heart. For the first time, I felt uneasy before my meeting with Tsering Norbu. What would he probably say? In a subdued mood, I finally trotted to his house.

The monk was naturally not at all surprised as I told him about my unhappy experience. "I expected this to happen. But I hadn't reckoned with it so soon. As I see, you have already opened yourself well for the prostrations."

Once again, I didn't understand anything. What could be so great about my frustration? However, Tsering Norbu didn't let himself become disconcerted. He pondered for a while until he had thought out an explanation: "Your pride stood in your way. It said to you: 'You don't need to subjugate yourself in front of anything or anyone.' Set your mind at ease. Most people from the West have this problem."

I defiantly contradicted him: "But that's alright. In front of whom should I subject myself? After all, I have enough self-respect."

"The two things have nothing to do with each other," the monk now smiled. "Do you believe that we Tibetans have no self-respect just because we practice the prostrations? Look at the people on the street."

It was true: These people truly radiated a healthy sense of self-worth. Nothing seemed phony about them, it streamed out naturally from within them.

Without waiting for a response, he continued: "The crucial point is this: to whom you bow is important. There are good spirits and evil spirits that you can attract through your veneration. You can entrust yourself to an angry demon or place yourself under the protection of loving gods. You must make this decision. In the prostrations, in any case, you venerate the qualities that you love, that are beautiful and worth striving for..."

I hadn't yet seen the exercises from this perspective. My reluctance now appeared presumptuous to me, and I was embarrassed. My teacher really had patience with me. Tsering Norbu acted like he didn't notice my self-conscious face. "We will talk about the qualities of this mental aspect in detail later. But for now, your experience of this morning is the topic at hand. It showed you that your pride stops you from opening up. For this reason, I want to tell you a story. It is about pride.

Look at that mountain."

The old monk pointed out of the window. I saw a mighty, broad mountain on the horizon. It was made of gray granite and completely barren. Spacious green meadows and fields spread out at its foot.

"The mountain is so exalted, Tsering Norbu continued. "It stands above everything else. Its walls are smooth and steep. Rain, as you know, is a symbol of fertility. Rain means growth and life. But how can a rainshower sink into the ground on a steep, exalted mountaintop? It naturally cannot do it at all since the water always runs off. You see: that is why that mountain over there rises to the heights barren and lonely. No fertile ground, in which flowers and bushes thrive, is formed on it. How different in contrast to it are the expansive, open valleys at its feet. The beneficial rainwater collects here. The lush meadows and forests grow there. Life and growth only take place in the valleys.

This is why I warmly recommend to you: do not be the proud mountaintop that stands unapproachable and exalted above everything else. No grass can grow on the heights. Come down and be a valley because it is there that you will receive the blessing of growth and fruitfulness. This is also the meaning of the prostrations: fruit can only thrive when you are open for the seeds."

Which seeds should these be? After the impressive image of the mountaintop, I was curious about this mysterious deeper level of the prostrations.

"Tell me about the inner path," I begged him. However, Tsering Norbu once again put my patience to the test.

"I am leaving tomorrow for a number of days. Go to the temple and practice more prostrations until I return. Forget your pride and concentrate only on the wave movement. As soon as I come back, we will talk about the inner nature of the exercise. It will very much enrich you, you will see! So, now I will pack my backpack and do some shopping."

Slightly aggravated, I walked back to the boardinghouse and got a sweater since the evenings had already become quite cool in autumn. Tsering Norbu had certainly already planned this trip some time ago, and he had just given me such short notice.

Soon afterwards, I could only laugh at my bad mood. Once again, I had taken myself too seriously. I had only known him for a short time and already thought he owed my explanations. How quickly we get used to things. Seen in retrospect, his pragmatic and simple way of telling me in short—typical for Tibetans—about his departure was completely appropriate.

While my friend was gone, I very much missed the conversations with him. The exercises once again were easy for me to do. My attack of pride disappeared as quickly as it had come, and it was pleasant to not have to think of anything while doing the prostrations. The wave-like harmony returned again.

The more the course of the movements became second nature to me, the more awake and lively I became in both the physical and mental sense. My body developed more resilience. The energy channels became increasingly free, and sensitive, powerful vital energy streamed through them. Through the alternating standing straight and lying flat, the body creates a bridge between the air and the Earth, the mind and matter.

My way of walking developed a cheerful sense of excitement, like a tree whose roots dig their way deeper and deeper into the earth while its crown stretches up into the heavens.

I noticed the quick improvement in my physical condition particularly during walks in the mountains. Now I could cross passes without any effort that I had only been able to master before by totally exerting myself. This naturally could also have been attributed to my increasing acclimation to the high-altitude region.

What Tsering Norbu had taught me up to now was an immense enrichment. There were so many new perceptions for me to take home with me. My thirst for knowledge, which had so plagued me at the beginning, gradually gave way to a pleasant sense of calm. I had the feeling that I had already comprehended the most important thing. Had I had any idea of the worlds into which Tsering Norbu still would initiate me, I wouldn't have been so relaxed.

Measured in terms of the quality of life that I had gained through my prostrations, the effort was insignificant: I only needed about ten minutes for these exercises. I wouldn't have any difficulty integrating this short period of time into my full everyday life at home.

Tsering Norbu finally stood at the door of my room one day. He was in the best of moods. "Hello, I'm back again. If you want, you can visit me this evening."

What a question! Full of joyful anticipation of our meeting, I bought incense sticks and a bag of barley flour for my friend. These were the traditional guest presents that I wanted to give him that evening.

I now knew that Tsering Norbu himself enjoyed instructing me about the prostrations and Buddhist philosophy. However, it was clear that his commitment didn't just apply to me in particular. Instead, he saw me as an empty vessel that wanted to be filled. He wanted to pass on a wealth of wisdom that addressed the spiritual needs of all people, independent of their culture. "In order to perceive the Buddhist view of life as being incisively correct, it makes no difference which culture you are a part of," remarked Tsering Norbu, "because it applies to all living beings."

"A person with a cheerful spirit can be happy. And happy people exercise a good influence on their surroundings," he had once explained. "Your mental and spiritual development should be based on two motivations: first, it will help you find your own joy in living. Then, the power of your inner satisfaction will emanate to other people." In this sense, he also wanted to create positive energies through his perceptions.

"Our world," he elaborated, "urgently needs such powerful people just as it needs powerful places. Without places of power, our Earth is threatened by mental, spiritual, and cultural demise. Societies that neglect such values risk their ruin. We need spiritual bearers of blessings for a healthy development of our Earth. This can be individual people, communities, or geographic power places."

Tsering was pleased about the presents I gave him that evening. He immediately lit an incense stick, which exuded its tart fragrance throughout the room. We made ourselves comfortable, and he told me a bit about his journey.

"I visited my old aunt. She became ill several weeks ago. Because she has no one, I had to take care of her. Now she is on the path to recovery. But that bus trip!" Tsering Norbu rolled his eyes. "We took one entire day. The streets were flooded, and the bus got stuck in ankle-deep mud. Didn't it rain here?" I shook my head. "In any case, I am happy to be here again. How have you been?"

With good will he listened to my enthusiastic report on the progress of the exercises. Yet, there was something I had to tell him. Just as spontaneously as some other decisions of the past weeks, I had reached a decision that afternoon.

"It is truly time to continue our teachings—someone is apparently bursting with curiosity here," smiled Tsering Norbu. But I didn't even listen to him.

"I have a surprise," now popped out of my mouth. How should I tell him the big news? Tsering Norbu made it easy for me. He looked at me in a calm and interested manner.

"I will stay here longer. I actually should go home next week. But I can't go yet."

Tsering Norbu didn't appear to be surprised: "Have you told the people at home?"

"Yes, I called before I came here. My boyfriend, the poor fellow, was rather annoyed. But I believe he understands.

"There is nothing else he can do with such an impulsive girlfriend like you," he grinned. So the matter was resolved. Sometimes it's good when no one asks questions. As seldom before in my life, it was clear as daylight to me that my chance to keep on learning so much about life was here at this place. And I wanted to make use of this opportunity. My everyday life was now too far away to create a bad conscience within me. I didn't even want to think of the business assignments that I had probably lost in the meantime.

"So," Tsering Norbu smiled in amusement, "then you are certainly ready for the inner path. Tomorrow I will tell you something about it. Most definitely! You can already come at 10 o'clock in the morning."

It was pitch-black as I walked home. I turned on my flashlight in order to avoid the potholes in the lonely alleys. The little town seemed to be totally dead. Just a few dogs howled at the moon, a narrow sickle in the heavens. Lights burned in just a few houses since most people had gone to bed early.

The Practice of the Yogis

The next morning I stood punctually at the door of Tsering Norbu's house. He was busy in the kitchen at the moment. "Do you even know how to brew buttered tea?" he called over to me while I took off my jacket.

"I've often watched," was my response.

"Then it is time for you to try it out yourself. After all, you should also learn something practical."

"Yes, I'd like to do that." He was just lifting a pot of black tea from the gas cooker.

"Look. Here is the cylinder." The monk got a round, 60-centimeter-long wooden cylinder from the corner and held it out to me. "Now fill the tea into it."

I wrapped a cloth around the hot handle of the pot and poured the steaming tea into the wooden cylinder.

"And now add a good piece of butter to it." Tsering Norbu handed me the bowl with the butter. "And salt. Go ahead and take two tablespoons, it doesn't hurt." I shook the salt into it and finally added a squirt of milk.

"So, that's it." The monk appeared satisfied. "Now mix everything together well."

I put a lid that had a wooden rod connected to it onto the cylinder, let the rod glide up and down so that the brew gurgled as it was mixed. After two minutes, Tsering Norbu made a sign for me to stop. "That's enough. Now you can pour the tea back into the pot."

"May I invite you to a pot of the most wonderful buttered tea?" I joked and poured two cups for us.

"Tastes good," praised Tsering Norbu. On the way to his chair, he drank an eye of butter with relish. "But now let us get started. I will first tell you something about the tradition of the prostrations.

Prostrations were propagated in Tibet with the introduction of Buddhism, which means this was about 1200 years ago. Do you know of any other exercise that is more than 1000 years old and has remained so popular up to this day that an entire folk practices it almost without exception?"

I shook my head. "That means that the prostrations must really be great."

"That is true. Prostrations cleanse the body and the mind, which is why many Tibetans make it into a regular ritual. There are astonishing stories of yogis and yoginis who live many years in lonely caves in order to achieve the highest level of perception. Do you know how their stories continue? Even in states of highest spiritual consciousness, which we call enlightenment, these people still practice these prostrations, naturally in addition to secret meditations and tantric exercises."

I wouldn't have thought this was true. A vague pride in being permitted to practice the same exercise as these spiritual yogis flooded through me. But I kept this feeling to myself. Tsering Norbu would have responded with that mocking-mild glance from the corner of his eye, which I could do without at the moment. As a modest person, he had little use for such presumptuousness.

It is the flowing movement of the wave that makes a prostration so unique. Tsering Norbu described it like this: "The greater part of our yoga exercises were assumed from the Indian yogas. Even Buddha lived with the Hindu yogis for many years in order to learn their practices. This is why the prostration contains all the yoga exercises. Put in other terms: the prostration is the essence of all yogas in a bud."

The monk had never before spoken of such dimensions. However, this thought was just as logical to me as it was interesting: yogis, who meditate on their seat-cushion from morning to night, must achieve some sort of compensation for their bodies. Prostrations were then ideal for restoring harmony to the body. Whether on a cushion in a cave or on an office chair in a modern company, the exercise is optimal for everyone who has too little physical compensation.

Yet, one question that I had long wanted to ask Tsering Norbu still burned in my soul: "Must I become a Buddhist in order to achieve the optimal effect from the prostrations?"

The monk calmly rejected the idea: "Not at all! You naturally do not need to be a Buddhist if you carry out this highest of all yogas. The Tibetan word for prostration is *chak-tsäl.* In translation this means the "veneration." In plain English: the prostration expresses a deep veneration. Because veneration goes beyond religion, anyone, no matter what his religious faith, can practice it."

"What is venerated?" I asked in curiosity.

"We Buddhists venerate the Buddha in a prostration. I do not mean the Buddha as a person here, but rather the virtues and good qualities that he represents. However, this is nothing for you at the moment. I have another suggestion: in the prostration, venerate something that you love and consider worth striving for. Simply imagine an object or a person for whom you show deep respect. And open your heart for this power. You will see: life becomes increasingly lovelier the more you open your heart."

It couldn't be that simple! Did the perception of happiness in life lie in such a plain bit of wisdom? The old monk simply replied: "Yes." I was perplexed.

"But," he continued, "do not just believe that everything is that simple. I want to say: Opening your heart is an easy exercise that will give you the highest degree of pleasure. The problem is only that we always set traps for ourselves that present us with trouble and suffering. This is why these moments of happiness are usually so short."

Why did everything have to be so complicated? What was the paradox that occurred so that the mind separated itself time and again from true happiness?

Tsering Norbu once again hindered my overzealousness: "A bit of Buddhist logic is necessary in order to understand this. More about it tomorrow.

Now I have a task for you again. It will intensify what we talked about a little while ago. The task is: When doing your prostrations tomorrow morning, open yourself up! While you stand in the starting position, say the following sentence: 'I open myself for all the beauty of this Earth.' Then repeat the following sentence with every prostration: 'I prostrate myself in the love of all beauty.'

This exercise," the monk continued, "is a wonderful beginning. And do not forget: in the prostration, your hands touch the three chakras of the top of the head, the throat, and the chest. Each chakra bears its own energy: by touching the top of the head, you connect yourself with the body of an enlightened being. The throat symbolizes enlightened speech. The enlightened mind is the heart.

We are naturally far removed from this ideal. But that does not matter since with the help of your exercises you will slowly approach it. And now enjoy your work."

I was still uncertain. "How should I open myself up? I have no idea how to do it," I protested.

Tsering Norbu remained hard: "Find it out for yourself. As I already said: true understanding does not happen through words, but through experiencing. So first be satisfied with my explanation and then wait to see what happens."

That night I sat on the terrace, wrapped in several sweaters and a blanket, and looked at the starry sky. Tsering Norbu was right: all people of this Earth search for happiness. That is probably the point that most connects all living beings with each other. Solely the way in which they want to fulfill their wishes and needs differentiates them. It may be attractive or repulsive—depending on what standards of values we set for ourselves.

Whether we feel friendship or rejection towards another human being also depends on this. The difference between rulers and subordinates, between victors and the conquered appears enormous in everyday life. Yet, the desire for personal happiness is the connecting link between all people. Of course, everyone fulfills this wish for himself according to his own standards. But how would it be if all people had the same concept of happiness? Ultimately, these goals are different from each other only because of ambition or some other nuances. Once a person has comprehended this point, it shouldn't be difficult to open up the heart. With this uplifting perception I was finally willing to go to bed.

The next morning at the temple was a total success. Even as I spread out my blanket for the prostrations, I had a pleasantly warm feeling around my heart. I directed my entire attention to this warmth, which slowly spread out. I mechanically moved my body up and down in a flowing motion. And into this wide space I spoke my sentence: "I open myself up for all the beauty of this Earth."

Now I no longer thought of anything. At some point, pictures of people who I had never liked surfaced. At this moment, I could even fully accept them. It was interesting that even these people were liked by their partners, children, and friends. Liking was then a matter of perspective. For a moment, I was able to turn off the categories of "likable" and "not likable."

When I had finished my round, I awoke from a state of deep trance. My heart spilled over with joy. I walked down the street to the market square. All these human beings suddenly became unique and worth loving. I smiled at each person I encountered—and received a smile in return. At this moment I could even like the street dogs whose yowling robbed me of my sleep at night. They just wanted to be happy as well.

The attentive boardinghouse landlady registered my state immediately. She held onto my arm as I wanted to go into my room and said: "The prostrations are doing you good. You are more balanced and relaxed."

I took a lukewarm shower and spent a comfortable afternoon on the terrace. I was very calm afterwards. I slowly began to comprehend what was happening to me: I was beginning to have a sense of well-being in my body. My mind was gradually moving away from its same old rut to strange, magical shores. It was like a summer rain that washed the dust from the streets.

Tsering Norbu showed himself less impressed by my lofty spiritual thoughts: "Only a fool lets himself be led up a garden path—first in one direction, and then in the other direction. And he must constantly chatter at the same time. As if his experiences were spectacular! Just yesterday you thought that you were not suitable for the exercises. Today you already believe that you have comprehended their essence."

He was silent for a moment. Then he considered backing up a bit: "You have decided on the prostrations. So do them. But stop judging every experience related to them. Register and observe everything, including your feelings. But do not constantly comment on them. Your mind almost goes head over heels in opening mental drawers and then closing them again.

Do not believe that this wonderful experience has changed your life. You were able to open up your heart one time, which is fine. It showed you that it is possible to do so. But this feeling will not last because you will have the tendency to close yourself time and again. This is why you must renew the opening of your heart day after day. Even so-called enlightenment is not permanent. Like all other perceptions, its source in your mind alone.

Oh, yes. By the way, with this we have already come to the topic of my instruction for today. Wait, I will first make a pot of tea."

I was glad that the monk was busy in his kitchen. His words had somehow hurt me. The truth is often hard to swallow. It was typical for Tsering Norbu that he didn't soften it in sweet milk but gave it to me plain. When he returned with the steaming pot of tea, I looked into his face. It was as warm and friendly as ever. I played a bit with a cookie in the teacup, squeezed the lukewarm tea out of it with my tongue, and chewed on it while lost in thought. Now and then I scribbled some notes in my book. When Tsering Norbu continued to speak, I was all ears once again.

"You wanted to know why people bring themselves suffering. Look at the everyday life of the people. How much worry and problems they carry around with them when things do not go according to their notions of them. They fixate their plans on pleasures and success because they understand this to be happiness. Then, at some point they discover: this so-called happiness is always just for a limited time. As soon as you hold it in your hands it always begins to slip away. A great love relationship may fade at some point. The terrific job soon turns into everyday routine. Even the nicest evening with friends also passes. As soon as these wonderful times are over, the feelings of elation quickly turn into sadness, disappointment, and anger."

"Why are human beings so shortsighted?" I wondered.

Tsering Norbu appeared to almost be sad. "Buddha gave the perfect explanation for this: our striving for this so-called happiness is distinguished by three mental poisons. These poisons are greed, hatred, and infatuation. With this, Buddha wanted to express: we are unhappy when our need for power, possession, or happiness goes unfulfilled. This is why we have an aversion against experiences that appear unpleasant to us. They simply do not fit into our idea of happiness."

"But that's normal. I'm also happy when I feel good or when I've reached a goal," I objected.

"How often do you live in this conscious, beautiful state? You spend most of your time organizing your present moment or making plans for the future. You plan how everything should be—and it should always be better than it is now."

It occurred to me that a girlfriend of mine once said the following sentence: "Happiness is the moments that I string like pearls on a chain. The times in between are an eternally long haul. It's absurd how much time and energy you devote in life for these few measly pearls!"

When I told Tsering Norbu about this, he had to laugh. "Your friend is completely right. In this small-minded striving for so-called happiness, people forget an important point: life trickles away minute by minute and flows towards death. This is why I warmly recommend that you use your time and enjoy the complete abundance of your existence in every second. Take life as it comes. Do not constantly chase after the pipe dreams that you want to achieve. As long as the mental poisons of greed, hatred, and infatuation determine how you act and feel, your mind will remain clouded. And you will never be able to enjoy the perfect quality of a moment.

Stop commenting about everything: 'This is good.', 'That is bad.', 'How ugly!', and 'Oh, how lovely. I want to have that.' You only feed your infatuation with this. You must see things as they are. Forget all expectations, and then you have nothing more to lose. True happiness namely consists of seeing things as they are. Then you can calmly devote yourself to the even stream of highs and lows."

"But how can I avoid getting caught in these traps time and again?" I replied despondently.

Now Tsering Norbu broke into peals of laughter. "Listen, why are you practicing your prostrations every morning? They are the path to opening your mind. Think about your experience this morning: As you walked through the market lost in thought, your heart was filled with everything you encountered. Wasn't this a moment of perfect openness? And this happened without you judging things and putting them into categories. You succeeded in cleansing and opening up your mind and heart with the prostrations."

At this point, someone knocked on the door of the house. Tsering Norbu interrupted himself to open it for the visitor. A neighbor was bringing by a bowl of apricots.

"My uncle just gave me a whole bag, and it's enough for

two people," he pushed his way through the door and comfortably sat down on Tsering Norbu's chair. The monk poured him a cup of tea.

"So you are the stranger in the city," the guest turned to me in Tibetan. My friend had to translate. "I have seen you frequently at the temple. Are you a Buddhist?"

"No, I'm not a Buddhist. But I find Buddhist philosophy fascinating and very logical." Tsering Norbu translated with a grin. "Besides, I very much like it here, and I like being here."

The neighbor was flattered and offered me an apricot. It was somewhat sour, but juicy and soft. I pulled out the pile of pictures from Germany that I always had with me and showed them to him. Photos of all types were very popular with Tibetans and always provided topics of conversation. He paged through the pictures of my parents, friends, the dog, and German churches with interest. It was at least a small gesture of cultural exchange.

The neighbor was talkative and then spoke about his own relatives, his married children, and the uncle with the apricots. The monk didn't have an easy job today!

I soon said good-bye. I later mused some more about the discussion with Tsering Norbu. You must cleanse your mind, he had said. But didn't our mind spontaneously express feelings? If this is true, then why should we fight against this spontaneity? I reminded myself of the morning: I could suddenly find people who were unlikable to be nice and briefly shed my aversion to them. This so-called spontaneity of emotion was then in no way spontaneous. It was apparently possible to change and manipulate it. Above all, it was very subjective.

This thought offered new perspectives. According to it, negative feelings originated from a personal, narrow-minded point of view. As soon as I looked beyond the rim of my hat, I would perceive new correlations. The only catch: the rim of one's own hat is much too familiar. I admit that I felt good within its limitations. But at the same time, I longed to expand these boundaries. What would Tsering Norbu probably say about that?

He didn't hesitate for a moment as I asked him about this the next day: "Expanding limitations has the precondition of cleansing the mind. Cleansing the mind, have you ever heard of this? Right now you are enthusiastic about how the prostrations refresh your body. You free the material of old waste substances and are glad when the organs and muscles function once again. That is wonderful. After all, your body should be a good home for you. Do not think that Buddhists disrespect their body.

But we say: the body is guided by the mind. Mind and body are a well-established team. I will give you one example: Had the mind not decided to do so, you would have never gotten into an airplane from Germany to Tibet. The body can only carry out what the mind orders. That is why the mind is the head of the house. The body is just his employee. When the boss is in a bad mood, he cannot instruct his employee as productively. Exactly the same thing happens with the body and the mind.

Most people think that they have to take care of just their bodies. The people in the West have an enormous physical culture! They are interested in chitchat, the newest fashions, the optimal clothing size, eccentric hairstyles, and clubs where people can increase the size of their muscles."

The old monk theatrically rolled his eyes upwards and waved his arms around wildly in the air. I had to laugh because he made such a funny figure. Today he was apparently aggressive and in the mood to provoke. For once I didn't contradict him since he was ultimately right. However, I found that the Tibetans were just as self-satisfied. Above all, the young fellows and women placed as much emphasis on their external appearance as we do. In the broadest sense of the word, this vanity could be categorized as courtship behavior, and that was normal after all. So there was no reason to run down the

West. But I didn't want to disturb Tsering Norbu's philosophical circles in any way and didn't interrupt as he continued in his agitation.

"The body culture goes even further. Think of your own apartment. I assume that you have a living room with comfortable arm chairs upon which a person can rest wonderfully. In the kitchen you cook food that you eat at the table in a cozy manner. Your bed needs good mattresses and a lovely blanket so that your body can relax well at night. You spend much time in the bathroom in order to clean yourself and make yourself beautiful. I will emphasize once again: all of this is important. Your body is your home, and you must therefore take good care of it.

But now we come to the critical point: what do you do to take care of your poor brain? It runs at high speed from morning to night. Even when the body rests, the brain ponders on this thing and that. How often do you plague yourself with sad and tormenting thoughts? Even at night your dreams often torment you with horrible images. When there is too much annoyance bottled up inside of you, it turns into poison.

Do you now understand why your mind also needs care? You must cleanse it from these negative tensions time and again. If you do not do this, your energy paths will become congested and prevent you from thinking clearly.

Every person desires to have a strong and pure mind. But without the proper care it will gradually grow weary, like a tool after years of use. This is why you must give as much loving care to your mind as to your body. You can achieve this with the help of the prostrations."

With this, Tsering Norbu ended his unusually long speech. I urgently needed a break. Just before I came, I had tracked down a bar of milk chocolate at the market. I now pulled it out of my pocket as a small reward for the both of us. After tearing open the foil, I generously offered Tsering Norbu a strip. As soon as he had put a piece in his mouth, he distorted his face. "Completely inedible!" He immediately spit it out. After more precise examination, the chocolate turned out to be covered with a grayish mold, which suggested the effect of heat over a longer period of time.

Not even the label "Made in Switzerland" could disguise the fact that the bar had probably traveled a long distance through India or southern China. Disappointed, I set the chocolate aside and once again reached for my notebook. Some questions about the formal course of the prostrations had occurred to me.

"What time of day is most beneficial for practicing the prostrations?" I asked Tsering Norbu. He was just rinsing out his mouth with buttered tea and cleared his throat again.

"The best time is in the morning after you get up. Your mind is clear and you greet the coming day. You should also do some prostrations in the evening in order to air your brain. Then you will not have any heavy dreams.

However, if you have no desire to do the usual prostrations in the evening, there is a variation: the so-called small prostrations. When you do these, you touch the floor only with your knees, forehead, and the palms of your hands. It is similar to the way Moslems bow towards Mecca."

"And what happens if I don't do any prostrations at all for a longer period of time?"

For example, when traveling on business I couldn't do my exercises in the hotel rooms. The table and bed hardly fit into these tiny chambers, not to mention extensive circular movements. Tsering Norbu's answer was strict. "Every interruption of your continuity is disadvantageous. When this happens, you stop the cleansing process in your body and mind. During your trips I recommend this: if the completely stretched-out prostrations are not possible, then practice some of the small prostrations every day." I was curious if at least this could be done in these small rooms.

What I didn't know at that time and learned only later at

a Buddhist center in Germany is that there is a further variation of the prostrations.

It works like this: after the starting standing position, touch the three chakras with the hands folded together, just as in the original version. Afterwards, first go down to the floor with the palms and then the knees. From this knee position, the hands slide a bit further forwards. This position now serves as a support in order to lay the upper body flat onto the ground. Now stretch out the hands completely to the front so that the entire body is stretched out on the floor. Stand up again in the reverse order. In this variation, the sliding-forward on the hands, as well as the circular movements of the arms before getting up, is omitted.

Later, I often practiced this exercise when there wasn't enough space or no sliding base was available for the classic large form. I consider it an acceptable compromise.

Visions

On one of these days, Tsering Norbu suggested: "Why don't you go visit Rinchen Pema? A change of air would do you good." I liked Rinchen Pema very much. She was Tsering Norbu's cousin and lived in a village, which could be reached with a bus ride of just a few hours. Whenever she was in the city, she stopped by to see her favorite cousin.

"You definitely have to come see me some time," she had always said to me, "you will like it where I live."

Rinchen Pema, a middle-aged woman, was somewhat suspicious about life in the city. She only came when she had important purchases to make. For example, when she needed fresh oil for the butter lamps of her house temple or wine-red cloth for her youngest son, who was also a monk. Otherwise, the family took care of its own needs for the most part.

The thought of visiting her appealed to me. I wanted a bit of a change. Besides, I had to agree with Tsering Norbu, who said: "After all, you are on vacation. You should travel around a bit."

Soon after this conversation, I packed a few articles of clothing into my backpack and walked to the market square. A public bus left from there twice a week for Rinchen's village. When I arrived, I asked some of the people working in the fields how to find the way to Rinchen's house. In the city, I hadn't noticed at all that the harvest was already in full swing. Between the golden-yellow stalks of barley in the fields, the colorful scarves of the women who cut the grain shone everywhere. It was a completely different world here without vehicles and the customary noise.

Rinchen Pema's house stood on a little hill, somewhat above the fertile farmland. The house was built of massive stone and plastered with brown clay. With its tiny windows, the building resembled a massive, impregnable fortress. I hesitantly walked up the steps. Since the wooden door was open, I entered and called her. The darkness in the long entrance hall with its many doors irritated me. At the same moment, Rinchen already came out of one of these doors. Beaming, she spread her arms: "What a surprise! Come in!"

She led me into a large kitchen. Rinchen Pema had been preparing lunch at the moment. Two cooking pots steamed on the giant cast-iron stove. Below, the flames licked at a pile of wood. In the long cabinet behind the stove, there was an orderly row of plates, teapots, and mugs for chang, a type of barley beer. A plastic tub stood in the corner, full to the brim with water.

"That is both our sink and our washroom," Rinchen laughed. "Since we have no running water in the house, we must always get the water from the stream behind the garden."

Next to the tub, I discovered a wooden stool with a few toothbrushes, soap, and two combs on it.

"You must certainly be thirsty." She got a glass from the cabinet, filled it with *chang*, and gave it to me. It tasted fresh and sweet. Fortunately, this brew wasn't strong since I hadn't drank any alcohol for weeks.

"It's nice that you came," she now said. "Unfortunately, I don't have much time at the moment. We are busy with the harvest right now. If you like, you can help. But you can naturally do whatever you please."

"I would like to help a bit," I responded spontaneously. To not have to think much for once was just what I wanted. The instruction by Tsering Norbu and all the thoughts that were turning the puzzle of my life inside out at the time were strenuous enough. I drank another glass of chang and then cut potatoes and carrots for the meal.

Soon afterwards, the entire family stormed in. I found Rinchen's husband likable at first sight. He was burly and had a clever face, into which the sun had tanned deep furrows. The four children, like organ pipes between ten and fifteen years old, threw their satchels into the corner as soon as the tempting fragrance of lunch reached their noses and sat down in front of the little dining tables. I was naturally the focus of attention while we slurped our vegetable stew from the tureens. The people here seldom got to see visitors from the West, let alone be permitted to entertain them as guests in their house. Full of pride, the children tried out their few English phrases on me.

"How are you?", "What's your name?", "How old are you?". Tomorrow they would have some things to tell at school! I immediately felt comfortable with them.

In the afternoon, I went out to the field with the entire family. Rinchen put a little crescent-shaped sickle in my hand and showed me how to cut the ears of grain. The harvest still was done with the traditional manual labor here. I couldn't discover a single tractor or any other type of modern farm equipment in the entire village. Now and then, curious neighbors came over to see me. They clapped their hands in enthusiasm when I was able to greet them in the Tibetan language: "Tashi delek." Unfortunately, the conversation came to an end at that point. It's good that Rinchen could speak a few words of English.

The unaccustomed squatting position while I cut the ears of grain soon made my legs stiff. Finally, Rinchen called me to take a break. We sat down in the shade of a tree and drank some glasses of buttered tea, into which we had sprinkled a handful of barley flour. I was dog-tired that evening.

"We sleep on the roof of the house during the warm season," Rinchen explained to me. "You can also sleep up there. But if it's too cold for you, stay in the kitchen."

I naturally preferred the roof. Between hay balls and sacks full of dried apricots, I unrolled my sleeping back on the roof of the house that night. Endless silence lay over the valley, with just a few crickets chirping. Before my leaden eyelids fell shut, a glistening shooting star shot across the sparkling sea of stars in the velvety black heavens. At that moment, there was nothing left for me to desire.

The next days melted into a kaleidoscope of natural occurrences. Fragrant grain tickled my nostrils. The transparency of the colorful mountain world, as if it were pinned on a canvas, sharpens the eyes. The sound of the stillness let my ears hear even the most delicate tones. Sometimes I was allowed to lead the yak to drink at the house stream. This hefty mountain of flesh trotted in a well-behaved way behind me on a rope while I concentrated on not slipping on the pebbles.

After five tranquil days, I wanted to go back to the city. I took leave of my friends and the yak. Rinchen put a bag of fresh vegetables, a piece of meat, and apricots in my hand with her best regards to Tsering Norbu. Before leaving, I took a picture of the entire family.

But the ride back was a catastrophe. When I returned to my room that evening, my nerves were worn to a frazzle. I had to talk to someone. I immediately went to Tsering Norbu in order to dispel my anger. I got so worked up in telling him my story that I accidentally poured the entire contents of the sugar jar on the floor.

"Now just don't get the idea of blaming other people for your anger," he giggled. "Now tell me one thing after the other."

It started with the bus being choked, full from the start, half of the village was apparently on the way to the city. I was naturally used to overfilled buses from my time in Asia, and the ride to the village hadn't been all that comfortable either. But having to stand in the central aisle, totally squashed in between countless people was simply too much.

The regular time of departure had long passed, but the bus driver waited for relatives who wanted to ride along. Finally, a women with her two children came. I have no idea where they found space, but the doors finally closed in any case. When we left with an hour's delay, I already had stiff limbs. And then the ride! We stopped at every farmhouse.

Almost every passenger wanted to take care of something on the way. A letter was brought here, and some vegetables were delivered there. Sometimes we just stopped so that someone could disappear into a house and briefly chat with friends. This cruise seemed to be never-ending.

But what was astonishing is this: while one person calmly did his errands, the others waited for him as cool as you please. Except for me, naturally. My mood had long reached rock bottom, and I punished the people with a scowl. How could they all radiate such good spirits in this overcrowded space?

"That is enough," Tsering Norbu interrupted my complaining at some point. "Now, what is the essence of this story?"

I tried to be objective. "Okay, I know. Everyone had something to take care of on the way. That's why they all were understanding about the others. It was just my bad luck that I wanted to get home as quickly as possible. But still," I insisted, "they could have hurried a bit more. Instead of three hours, we needed six."

"Too much for you. Do you know that so-called reality actually does not exist?"

My mood was too bad right now to talk about philosophy with Tsering Norbu. Besides, there wasn't anything that could be changed about it anyway.

However, my teacher remained stubborn. Every unpleasant situation was a welcome occasion for him to contemplate the nature of the mind.

"What I mean is that there is no ultimate reality," he kept on. I admitted defeat, grabbed a glass of lemon water, and let myself fall onto one of the chairs in a cross-legged position.

"I'm all ears," I now grinned. "So what went wrong?" The sheer presence of Tsering Norbu could lift my spirits.

"Let us summarize: All of the passengers in the bus experienced the same situation. It naturally is not true that everyone had errands to do. It certainly was not even the half of them." I nodded involuntarily. One tends sometimes to exaggerate.

"That means that some passengers had just as little advantage from the delay as you did," Tsering Norbu continued. "Yet, they remained in a good mood. The secret is: They made the best out of this situation and let themselves feel good. At the same time, you put on a black face in frustration just because the journey did not correspond with your notions. You got stuck on your idea of how reality should be. And you made yourself unhappy.

The opposite applied to the others: They simply adjusted to the unavoidable situation and remained satisfied. Do you see how people can live in different realities?"

"How does that go?" I asked at a loss.

"By creating a pleasant reality for yourself. This is quite simple: be the doer and not the victim."

Tsering Norbu had hit on a sore point here. How often I had felt myself totally at the mercy of situations in which I could only react with helplessness and anger.

"You could have concentrated on other interesting things related to this trip," the monk continued. "Why didn't you more closely observe your fellow travelers or study the colors of the mountains? You could also have meditated or paid attention to your breathing. You see: there are always a number of possibilities in order to master a situation. You chose the worst possibility.

Let me give you a tip: as soon as the black energy is created inside of you, immediately exhale it. Exhale it until it has completely disappeared. By doing this, you will avoid being filled to the brim with annoyance. Then concentrate your mind on pleasant and interesting things. Inhale these energies as bright light. You will see: every situation in life contains a number of aspects at the same time. Which aspect you make a part of you is up to you. The most important thing is that you alone are responsible for the happiness in your life. So reject your role of victim and become a person who shapes her own life."

Verses for Those Who Practice

How quickly the time slipped by! After a look at the calendar one day, I determined in astonishment that I had been here for three months. This inconspicuous place, which at first had just been meant to be an inconvenient stopover and was never my goal, had in the meantime become so dear to me that I almost felt at home here. The morning prostrations and the instruction by Tsering Norbu had long become a solid part of my everyday life.

In addition, I had also made friends with some nice people in the course of the weeks, like a Tibetan couple who was about my age. Sometimes they invited me to dinner, and I talked with them in my few bits of broken Tibetan. We laughed for hours at banal things. Now and then I helped Sönam, the woman, prepare the meal. It was fascinating to see the unbelievable imagination with which she could work barley, the basic food of Tibet, into such a great variety of dishes. Then we sat in her dark kitchen in front of the giant stove and plucked dough cakes into boiling water. Karma, her husband, spun wool or looked after the goats in the meantime. Karma owned a little store in the old part of town. With this income, a vegetable garden, and some goats, he and Sönam got by fairly well.

My acquaintance with the Chinese Chao Li was a thorn in the side for my Tibetan friends. After all, the Chinese were simply considered "members of the occupying forces" in the eyes of the Tibetans. But Chao Li was alright. He was a teacher and had been transferred to Tibet on orders. His family lived far away in southern China, and he had to endure here all alone.

"I don't like it at all in Tibet," he sometimes complained. "At best I'd like to go home immediately, to my wife and my daughter. But my established post is here. Politics? They don't interest me one bit. As far as I'm concerned, the Tibetans can have their independence. Even we Chinese are only a toy for

Peking and have to subject ourselves to its restrictive government."

Since Chao Li spoke English quite well, I liked to discuss the situation in the country in detail with him.

One day I received a letter from Germany. My partner in life missed me very much. As I read his lines, I felt a great ache around my heart. I also sensed a yearning. Autumn had long come to Tibet, and the nights became severely cold. Sometimes there was already ice on the water puddles in the morning. It had become time for me to go back home. Just as intuitively as I had extended my stay three months ago, I booked a return flight that day. I had to be in Lhasa in one week.

Tsering Norbu wasn't surprised by my decision. "It is good for you to go home again. However, before your departure there are some things that I will teach you. Because of this, we will make intensive use of the remaining time."

We spent long afternoons with each other during this week. Sometimes the old monk told stories of the great yoga masters of Tibet. Even in the bitter-cold months of winter, some of them only wore very thin clothing made of cotton. Every normal person who did this would certainly have frozen. But thanks to tantric rituals, these Grand Masters created so much inner heat within their bodies that they lived through the cold without harm. Tsering Norbu explained a bit about the practice of their meditations, and translated some philosophical texts and wonderful poems that they had written in their caves. I was particularly fascinated by the yogi Milarepa. Even today, every Tibetan schoolchild knows his famous verses by heart.

However, an important part was still missing for me to carry out the prostrations completely. Until now I had always recited the saying: "I prostrate myself in love of all beauty." This sentence had triggered a feeling of well-being within me and a strange sense of fearlessness at the same time. But the

Tibetans recited substantially longer verses when they practiced. What visions did they create with them?

One afternoon, Tsering Norbu was willing to initiate me into these complete recitations. "Today I will give you the essence for the perfect cleansing and motivation of the mind. It will sensitize and open your chakra points.

The text may sound unusual for you at the start, perhaps too abstract or pathetic. But have trust in these verses and memorize them well. They are perfect.

The great yogis since time immemorial have recited precisely these verses. They helped them achieve physical well-being and mental perfection. In the same way, they will also be of use to you."

After this introduction, he added: "Mind you: the following rituals are suited for people who are familiar with the spiritual ideas. You will also be familiar with these soon. I have prepared some texts for you that will lead you there. I will also say them for you after this. But first listen to our classic recitation that we Tibetans practice."

"Before we start with the prostrations, we speak the Buddhist refuge formula three times:

'I take refuge in Buddha.

I take refuge in Buddha's teachings.

I take refuge in the community of those who practice.'

During the prostrations, we imagine the figure of the Buddha in his 35 different manifestations. Each of these manifestations reflects another one of the Buddha's qualities or virtues. With each prostration, we recite one of the following verses. One 'round' is therefore 35 prostrations.

1.
Into the enlightened teacher Buddha Shakyamuni
I prostrate myself.

2.
Into Buddha, who destroys all illusions,
I prostrate myself.

3.
Into Buddha, who is the radiant light of a jewel,
I prostrate myself.

4.
Into Buddha, who fights all the evil spirits,
I prostrate myself.

5.
Into Buddha, who leads all brave warriors,
I prostrate myself.

6.
Into Buddha, who embodies the greatest bliss,
I prostrate myself.

7.
Into Buddha, who radiates sparkling fire,
I prostrate myself.

8.
Into Buddha, who radiates sparkling moonlight,
I prostrate myself.

9.
Into Buddha, the sight of whom brings perfect insight,
I prostrate myself.

10.
Into Buddha, the sparkling moon,
I prostrate myself.

11.
Into Buddha, who is without a flaw,
I prostrate myself.

12.
Into Buddha, the generous giver,
I prostrate myself.

13.
Into Buddha, the pure being,
I prostrate myself.

14.
Into Buddha, the bearer of deepest purity,
I prostrate myself.

15.
Into Buddha, the divine ocean,
I prostrate myself.

16.
Into Buddha, the divine being of the divine ocean,
I prostrate myself.

17.
Into Buddha, the wonderful kindhearted one,
I prostrate myself.

18.
Into Buddha, the fragrant sandalwood,
I prostrate myself.

19.
Into Buddha, the endless splendor,
I prostrate myself.

20.
Into Buddha, the immense light,
I prostrate myself.

21.
Into Buddha, who is perfectly without cares,
I prostrate myself.

22.
Into Buddha, the son of the content one,
I prostrate myself.

23.
Into Buddha, the radiant blossom,
I prostrate myself.

24.
Into Buddha, who enjoys the radiate light of clarity
and thereby comprehends reality,
I prostrate myself.

25.
Into Buddha, who enjoys the radiant light of the lotus
and thereby comprehends reality,
I prostrate myself.

26.
Into Buddha, the overflowing abundance,
I prostrate myself.

27.
Into Buddha, the perfect circumspection,
I prostrate myself.

28.
Into Buddha, whose name is most highly respected,
I prostrate myself.

29.
Into Buddha, the king who holds up the flag of victory
above the senses,
I prostrate myself.

30.
Into Buddha, the glorious one
who completely overcomes all illusions,
I prostrate myself.

31.
Into Buddha, who is victorious in all battles,
I prostrate myself.

32.
Into Buddha, the glorious one
who has realized perfect self-control,
I prostrate myself.

33.
Into Buddha, the glorious one
who allowed the outer world to be created,
I prostrate myself.

34.
Into Buddha, the jewel lotus who has overcome everything,
I prostrate myself.

35.
Into Buddha, the complete enlightened one,
the great jewel in the lotus, the king
who rules the mountains,
I prostrate myself.'"

Tsering Norbu had recited these verses in a soft and absorbed way. I listened, fascinated by this abundance of unfolded visions in front of my inner eye. Now the monk looked calmly at me.

"Perhaps you are astonished that every verse begins with 'in Buddha' instead of 'in front of Buddha.' The text would be properly translated in both cases. But I think the sentence 'in front of Buddha' implies a spiritual separation: here is the great Buddha—there I am, a small human being. On the other hand, with 'in Buddha' you connect yourself into unity with Buddha. These words express that Buddha is a part of you in all of his aspects."

We needed a break. Oblivious to everything around him, Tsering Norbu took his little prayer-wheel in his hand. It rotated squeakily while the monk softly murmured the mantra "Om Mani Padme Hum—Oh, you jewel in the lotus blossom." He appeared to still dwell completely in the verses. In the meantime, at the gas cooker I made an effort to brew some sweet tea with milk. As soon as I returned with two full cups, he once again picked up the thread.

"I have given much thought to how these verses of life philosophy can be made understandable for Western people. Their meaning and effect should naturally remain the same. A short time ago, I spoke with two other Lamas about this. Both had also spent a longer period of time in America and have understood your mentality quite well. We finally achieved a satisfactory result. Listen well:

I prostrate myself into the love of all living beings.

I prostrate myself into endless patience.

I prostrate myself into absolute honesty.

I prostrate myself into compassion for the poor.

I prostrate myself into absolute tolerance.

I prostrate myself into radiant truth.

I prostrate myself into deep circumspection.

I prostrate myself into true kindness.

*I prostrate myself into the golden abundance
of all encounters that this unique day
will give me."*

I quickly wrote down the verses in my notebook. When Tsering Norbu had finished speaking, I repeated the recitations. I let each verse melt in my mouth. How odd: words like circumspection, kindness, or honesty sounded rather unaccustomed to the ear since they are gradually dying out in our language. Was it only in our language or also in our consciousness? I somehow found it soothing to speak these words. There is an old truth: feelings and values are only distinguished through words. An example: as long as I speak negatively about a person, my heart will hardly warm up for him. If I describe this same person with warm, friendly attributes, it's easier for me to like him. Or, in other terms: everything only has the value that I attribute to it.

Related to the recitation, this means: when I consciously speak of a positive quality, it gains in power and can become a valuable treasure.

I was still pleasurably mumbling the verses as it dawned on me how precisely the Lamas had chosen these virtues.

Tsering Norbu said of this: "Our age urgently needs instruction in honesty, circumspection, patience, and kindness. Otherwise, there is the danger that our hectic striving for success and pleasure will eat us up. I suggest we call them 'Verses for Western People Who Practice'."

"What is the most appropriate way to recite them?" I wanted to know.

"I have given you nine verses. They are the basic foundation for your future practice.

It is optimal for you to think in a cycle of ten. To the nine verses, add one more esteemed value that is important to you at the moment. At the same time, you can add another esteemed value every day. But it can also be the same one each time. It depends on your preferences.

You can also prostrate yourself mentally before flowers, trees, or people that you respect. What you would like to recite is up to your desire and your imagination. As you see, there are so many possibilities of refreshing your motivation. There are no limits set for the esteemed values. So, now I have a present for you."

A present for me? I looked questioningly at Tsering Norbu.

He searched through a pile of papers on the table, from which he pulled out an envelope.

"I have already been keeping this for some time now. The day has come today."

He took two written pages out of the envelope. A text was written on them in curved Tibetan calligraphy.

"These," he explained, "are the 35 prostrations. I have written them down for you. It doesn't matter if you cannot read them. They have their own power."

How much effort this monk had made with me! I carefully packed the envelope into my pocket. I would always honor it.

In my room later on, I wrote the nine verses in various colors on a piece of paper. On the outside border, I drew some decorative motifs. Then it was more enjoyable to learn the lines by heart. The next morning, I discovered with amusement that a great many esteemed values of my own occurred to me without any effort.

Despite the feeling of happiness about this newly discovered treasure-chest, I was melancholy. The departure was just around the corner, and I had to take leave of my friends. We celebrated some happy parties with each other on these evenings, at which chang naturally was always present. So I went to my morning activities at the monastery somewhat later than usual.

I coincidentally met Tsering Norbu on the street in the afternoon. We only saw each other sporadically at that time since I was busy with the preparations for my departure.

"I have one more little lesson for you before you go," he said. "Do you have time this evening?"

Tsering Norbu naturally had precedence over any other appointments. When I later knocked on the door, he was already expecting me.

"I want to round off my instructions of the last hour. Then you will be perfectly prepared for your practice at home.

As you already know, the cycle of ten determines your

exercises. I would like to give you two more variations, both of which are very helpful.

One variation is the following: once a week you recite all ten esteemed values according to your own wishes. It doesn't hurt if there are qualities among them from the 'Verses for Western People Who Practice.' But, in principle, you should spontaneously think them out for yourself. Either write down the verses before the prostrations and then read them, or let the esteemed values flow out of you intuitively during the prostrations. With the help of this exercise, it will become clear to you which esteemed values are of particular significance for you. Once you have tried them out, you can better integrate them into your everyday life.

Here is the second variation: Definitely recite, also once a week, the original Tibetan prayer with the 35 verses. The text may sound curious, but it leaves positive traces in the subconscious. Have deep trust in these verses and remember: they have already helped countless people achieve physical and mental harmony. This is why the verses will also have an effect within you." In conclusion, this wonderful monk gave me one more valuable piece of advice to take with me: "Always be aware: all the positive qualities that you speak of in the prostrations lie within you. Only your clouded mind stops you from realizing them. This means that you do not put on anything foreign with the prostrations. To the contrary, you develop your true, personal strength with their help. You will not become another person but solely come closer to your own personal nature. I am happy that you have the courage to walk this path. It will open your eyes to deeper wisdom."

Then he also added: "Always remember that everything that glows does not come from somewhere outside of you. To the contrary, it has long been concealed within you. You only need to unearth it like a long-forgotten treasure. And now go your own way. I wish you a good journey."

My friend waved at me a long time in parting. We both knew that I would soon return.

Little Devils of the Mind

During the first days of my return, Germany passed by me like a film. Although I had seen this film often enough and was familiar with the individual scenes, there was a screen separating me from the plot. Often I sat there and observed all these boring pictures. I was suffering from culture shock. This condition continued for some days before I could finally enter through the screen into what was happening around me. My joy in living gradually returned as well.

I energetically went to work on setting up my new exercise area. While I was walking around our lovingly furnished rooms without a clue, the golden words of my friend Tsering Norbu occurred to me: "These dwellings are solely designed for physical comfort!", he had once said in reproach. How right he had been! A couch then wandered into the classified ads of our local newspaper so that a corner would be free in my favorite room.

From the first moment, I felt good in this new spot. A window looked to the east, where the morning sun would shine in while I practiced my yogas. I set up a little ritual table that I decorated with a shiny red scarf. On this table I draped objects that I was fond of. First there was the chestnut from a friend's garden. He had given it to me that autumn before he emigrated to Australia. Then there was a donkey's horseshoe. I had once found it during a journey through the north Indian Himalayas. The horseshoe was lying close to a house into which I had moved for several days. Even afterwards, I had never been certain whether my tender romance with the interesting Englishman, who I had met there, had something to do with the horseshoe. The black feather from a magpie also came from the same period. The main figure on my ritual table was naturally the little Buddha figure of bronze. Chao Li, my Chinese friend, had given it to me on the way home:

"It is a talisman and power object," he had said. "Take good care of it."

I finally bought a thin wool blanket for my knees. I had brought along the two wine-red pieces of linen for my hands from Tibet since I would keep on using them. The verses were on two sheets of paper: on one, the original prayer of the 35 Buddhas and the nine esteemed values on the other. Now I was ready. But an obstacle came up with which I hadn't reckoned: the brand-new, cuddly velour carpet that enveloped the entire room in a warm yellow-ocher. How was I supposed to glide forwards on it? It was impossible with my pieces of cloth. Did I have to set up "my corner" somewhere else in the apartment? After another ramble through the house, I could find no other larger area with a smooth floor.

Floors made of wood, marble, tiles, or linoleum would have been perfect. But our rooms all had carpets. The problem soon took on interpersonal dimensions: with an unpleasant growl as an undertone, my partner refused to leave the good ocher-yellow carpet to the classified ads, as I had suggested in my overzealousness. He, a patient person by nature, became stubborn on this point. I had to think of something else. Good advice was dear in this case. Tsering Norbu was hardly out of range, and now the problems were starting.

I soon had an idea. My solution was quite simple and practical. At the do-it-yourself store I purchased a piece of stiff linoleum. I cut it to the dimensions of 2.5 x 2 meters and spread it out on the floor. At the corners, I weighed it down with bricks. It didn't look very elegant, but that didn't bother me. When I was done with the exercises, I could roll it up and put it in the corner.

Although the matter of the carpet had delayed the go-ahead for my rituals by two days, it hadn't detracted at all from my motivation. I was curious about the effect of my exercises on my everyday life in Germany! Despite this, or perhaps because of it, I initially kept it a secret that I practiced the prostrations in accordance with the old saying: don't count your chickens before they hatch.

No one, except for my partner, naturally, heard anything about my morning yoga at first. But it didn't last long until I told friends about it. Or in more precise terms, I had to tell them about it.

Everyone soon noticed that a change had happened within me since I came back from Tibet. Clients with whom I had worked for years were amazed that I had suddenly become a relatively poised person—a quality with which I had never adorned myself before. Friends wondered about my composure when they appeared late for a date or when the evening at the movies turned out to be a flop. That I was more slender than before naturally became conspicuous, particularly to the women. Even my partner, who was usually skeptical about any type of "esoteric stuff," as he called it, supported my development. No wonder—it was also to his advantage: our home atmosphere had become more harmonious than ever before and petty bickering became unnecessary. This change didn't occur because I halfheartedly gave in when a quarrel threatened to break out, as I had done in earlier times. On the contrary, I rested so calmly and pleasurably in my own center that I no longer lost my emotional equilibrium right away. Tensions didn't even have the chance to develop.

What an effect a cleansed body and fresh mind have! I actually felt much younger. It was clear that every "vacation effect" after a wonderful trip continues for a time. But everyday life normally gets the upper hand at some point, and the old habits creep back in. That's why the people who knew me were quite irritated.

"What is actually going on with you?" Ingrid probed after a few weeks and several glasses of wine. "I only know you to be like that when you've fallen in love. Have I missed out on something important?"

"You smartie, how did you find out about it? I actually have fallen in love," I giggled.

"You did *what*? With a Tibetan?"

"Certainly not. For once, with myself."

Ingrid's questioning look amused me, and I blurted it out straight-away. I now told her about my new practice. Ingrid listened with interest, and the same evening I had to perform several prostrations for her. The practice later reached more people, and other friends also began to do the ritual of the prostration.

The integration of my practice into everyday life was more simple at first than I had expected. I got up fifteen minutes earlier in the morning and took a few deep breaths at the open window. Then I was ready for the yoga. I started my day fresh and with an open heart.

In the hectic of the morning, where every moment was precious, I was thankful for the effectiveness of this exercise. To this day, I don't know of any other yoga that produces the same result in so few minutes. In Tibet, where I had had all the time in the world, this had never consciously occurred to me.

The exchange of letters with Tsering Norbu remained lively. I missed him very much, and his letters were extremely valuable to me. I didn't know of any comparable wise man in Germany and longed for discussions on spiritual topics.

The most burning question I had was still: How was it possible for the body and mind to become as refreshed as I was now experiencing?

An explanation traveled with the mail for many weeks. Finally, I held the letter in my hands. Tsering Norbu had responded extensively, naturally with Buddhist reasons. While I read his lines, I imagined how he sat next to the petroleum lamp in his room, a piece of paper in front of him, and carefully searched for the appropriate words. I remembered how he always attentively looked at me during our conversations to see if I was following him. After four pages, some things were more clear to me.

He wrote: "Buddha said: Things are guided by the mind. This means that everything you experience and live through initially comes from your mind. Experiences and thoughts were already within you before you experienced and thought them. This is why things will only happen to you that your mind can also accept.

I will give you an example: When you were a child, perhaps your teachers and parents continually told you that you could not draw. They possibly saw one of your drawings and thought it did not turn out well. As a result, you stored the information of 'I cannot draw' in your head. Even later as an adult you never again picked up a colored pencil—and all of this just because you had been programmed in this respect since your childhood."

Furthermore, Tsering Norbu wrote: "As you know, the mind is practically the boss of the body and gives it guidelines. This is why it depends on you which information you feed your mind. This leads me to the answer to your question: According to conventional ideas, your body with all of its functions and organs must age within a certain period of time. As long as you believe in the compulsive deterioration of the body, this will happen. Yet, if you let go of these negative expectations, your body's aging process will then slow down. Your mind merely has to change the image of your self. Imagine that you are young and your body is dynamic and full of resilience. You should therefore combine this idea of a flexible body with your practice of the prostrations and then you will achieve the optimal results."

I put the letter aside for a moment and imagined the old monk. Despite his 75 years, he seemed supple and youthful. In fact: He was the best example for the truth of his statement. An interesting comparison for this occurred to me: In one sense, computers are comparable to the human mind. A com-

84

puter carries out a command according to a given program. If I no longer need this program, I can put it into the "wastepaper basket" with a click of a key. Now there is room for another program corresponding to the new tasks. Translated to the mind, this means: I can get rid of old concepts that have become superfluous and store new ideas in their place.

It was interesting how Tsering Norbu connected with this idea in the course of the letter. He wrote: "If, since your childhood, you have believed that you cannot draw, toss this idea out of your head. If you feel the desire to draw, sit down today and start with it. Uplift yourself with the sentence: I can draw. The same principle functions with the physical feeling. If you have thought up to now that your body is inflexible, throw this thought out of your mind as well. You will automatically move in a more supple manner. Let me emphasize once again: the mind is the boss in the body, and the body will be oriented according to the mind's idea.

I am not talking about wonders here. There is naturally no person, even with the strongest faith, who is immortal. Every bit of matter is part of the cycle of growth and decay, and it is good so. But, with these exercises, you can slow down the process of aging—as long as your mind and body work together. The mind is namely more receptive and flexible than you believe it is capable of being. It just wants to be challenged. Your body feels younger at the moment because your mind is balanced. For this to continue in the long term, you must reorient your ideas in the way that I have just explained to you."

At the close of his letter, Tsering Norbu added: "Definitely keep on practicing the prostrations. Feed your visions with positive pictures. Openness and love of all the beauty of this Earth will then develop on their own."

The months flew by. In the corner where I practiced, I always placed a bouquet of fresh flowers. The photograph of a

Himalayan mountain chain hung on the wall—a touch of the infinity of all being.

My exercises always put me in a great mood, and I felt better than ever before. Because my mind was clear, the work at the computer was relatively easy for me. I slept one or two hours less at night and therefore finally had time to do all the things for which the energy had previously been lacking. Sometimes I took extended excursions through the city with the camera, photographed people and house corners. I took a great many snapshots of our cat. I developed my work with endless patience in the new darkroom that I had set up in the cellar. Everything was optimal.

Until the day I had no desire at all to carry out the practice that I had so loved before. The attack came as quickly as the one back in Tibet, where it was my pride that had stood in my way. Now I had difficulty in reciting. I spent my days in discontent and was no longer satisfied. I didn't understand the world anymore. Naturally: there had been times before when I sometimes didn't have any desire to practice. The bed was simply too cozy! But as soon as I had overcome this inner lazybones and stood in front of my ritual table, the prostrations had always inspired me. But now a true crises was at hand.

Tsering Norbu didn't waste many words on my lamentations in his responding letter. Buddhists just don't judge emotions to be as final as we do. Everything is in the process of growing and decaying. He called my aversion a "little imp."

"It is very clear," he wrote, "that your imp wants to return to his old patterns of behavior. He wants his beloved standards once again because they are so comfortable and familiar to him."

This imp was really fresh. While I practiced as mechanically as a clock, he sneered in my ear: "I don't want to be generous. I also don't want to open up my heart." Nothing could get him down.

"Do not be all that hard on him," Tsering Norbu suggested. "And do not chase him away in haste. The imp is namely a part of you. He is the old ego that you looked after for so long. Habits only fade away slowly. You cannot and should not erase them from one day to the next."

And further: "If your aversion against breathing in the golden light of such virtues (his writing was sometimes quite corny) becomes too strong, take a break. If you are angry at a friend, then accept this anger. Do not ignore it by acting meek. But also do not feed it by lending this talkative imp your ear."

My eyes were caught by the next sentence: "With this we have reached one deep meaning of Buddhism. You do not need to suppress negative feelings by putting a bell jar of holiness over yourself. This is not Buddhism. Buddhism means savoring deep joy and enjoying openness. If you practice persistently, such pleasant moments will become intensified and even more extensive in the course of time."

At the end of this letter, Tsering Norbu added the following advice: "At the moment you should return to the most simple exercise that I taught you on the first day. Do you remember? Return to your body, feel the movement of the great wave, and enjoy its rhythm. Recite nothing while you do this. This will do you good and let your circling thoughts come to rest. Exert yourself until your heart beats more quickly and you get out of breath. The prostrations can unburden you in the same way as a run in the woods. If you are tired enough, your aggressions will go up in smoke and your mind will become refreshed."

It turned out that the old monk was right. Soon I once again savored the prostrations in all their variations. Above all, I developed a feeling for what might do me good at the moment. Before I started my practice session, I listened within myself for a moment. In this way, I found out which variation would be especially helpful now.

During the course of time I trusted increasingly in the standard Tibetan version of the 35 Buddhas. Tsering Norbu had naturally hit the nail on the head with his advance warning that these odd descriptions could be irritating at the start. But he had also advised: "Do not think much about it. Simply recite the verses. You will see that they exert a secret power over you."

This was actually true: The more frequently I spoke these words, the more they sank into the finest body channels as a filigree energy. I had the feeling that these 35 verses contained all the aspects of a perfect personality and observed how the magical power of these words awakened an unknown feeling of self-assurance within me.

The seed lies concealed deep within the soul of every human being. It only waits to be discovered. With the "yoga essence in a bud," I was now certain that I held the key to this unimagined potential in my own hands.

Golden Breath

Before I knew it, spring had returned to the land. With the first delicate rays of sunshine, a quiet longing for the strong blue of Tibet's skies arose within me. During the winter, I had already secretly made arrangements for the next trip, but this time only five week's vacation was the definitive limit. I couldn't afford to go for months without earning any money again.

As soon as the wheels of the airplane hit hard on the ground of the familiar Tibetan highlands, I had a warm feeling around my heart. While the other passengers rushed quickly into the heated reception hall, I remained standing outside in the cold morning for a moment. The air streamed sharp and clear up my nose. The snow-covered mountain ranges seemed close enough to touch. When the machine finally turned off its droning engines, there was a perfect silence above this white plateau for the span of one breath. Just a donkey squealed in a heartrendering way like a leaky machine somewhere.

I was surprised at how much I had missed this solitude during the past months. I took another deep breath of this fresh morning air and then entered the hall as the last passenger. A pile of formulas were waiting to be filled out at the arrival counter.

Since it took several days to reach my little town by bus, I wanted to start off the next morning. I wasn't in a hurry and enjoyed the familiar sound of snatches of Tibetan conversation that I picked up while hauling my luggage through the streets of Lhasa.

At a hotel, I dug out a few scraps of Tibetan and asked for a room: "Nga la kangpa chik go kyi yö." The porter's bored look immediately brightened up. A foreigner who spoke Tibetan! He showered me with a flood of words that ended with a questioning look. That's what I got for showing off, I naturally didn't understand a word of it. The porter also seemed to be disappointed. He formally handed me my key. Once again,

I got up the courage to ask him about a restaurant. I now had a huge hunger for a bowl of thukpa, Tibetan noodle soup. "Sakang kawa yo re?"

Without a word, the porter pointed to the street and bent his index finger to the left a moment later. I would have also understood that in Tibetan.

A trip in Tibet is strenuous and time-consuming. In a small bus, wedged in between thick wool coats, bobble hats, and sacks of potatoes, it takes at least twice as long. Every once in a while, when my neighbor bent forwards to swipe a handful of tsampa from his travel bag and stick it in his mouth, I got a brief glimpse at the passing steppe landscape. There are high points in life in which you would like to stop time. In other situations, it's a mercy when it does trickle by, and so the end of the road finally came at some point. I sorted the various parts of my body into the position meant for them and jumped in relief into the open.

The usual bustle prevailed at the market square. Streams of people squeezed through between the stands. Those who had come from further away pulled mules behind them on which they had packed their goods. After a long, bitterly cold winter, these people were glad to see the first warming rays of sunshine that finally announced the coming of spring. Shivering, I pulled up the collar of my parka while I pushed through the tumult in the direction of my old familiar boardinghouse. On the way there, familiar faces emerged with bright greetings: "Tashi Delek, aja!" floated towards me. How many people with whom I had never spoken before sent me a smile of recognition!

The woman farmer from whom I had always bought my fruit the year before slipped me a handful of dried apricots. "Welcome, my friend." I picked a little stone and a few dried blades of grass out of the shrunken apricot and put it in my mouth. The apricot was as hard as a bonbon, and I chewed on it a bit until it reluctantly released its fruity sweetness.

My friendly landlady later prepared a giant pot of steaming buttered tea for me in the kitchen. Three big cups of it reconciled me with the exertions of the journey. Now I was back home again.

But the biggest surprise came from Tsering Norbu. "I have been waiting for you," he declared casually as I stood in front of his door a short time later with a bag of tsampa and some yak butter. I hadn't gotten used to the thin air yet, and just the few steps to his place had caused me to be out of breath. I thankfully sank down onto a chair. Tsering Norbu was busy at the moment with the chest in the corner, sorting prayer sheets.

"I will be done right away," he said. "Go ahead and rest a bit." But I followed him. I was both disappointed and curious: "You couldn't possibly know that I was coming," I probed. After all, I hadn't announced my intentions of visiting him. Now the nice surprise was ruined.

He blinked at me in a profound and wise way: "I simply knew it." But he began to giggle the next moment. He gave me a friendly pat on the shoulder: "You are still the same old person. Always wanting to know everything down to the last detail. That reassures me very much." Did his premonition come from a deeper intuition that couldn't be explained?

That evening, we didn't get caught up in philosophy. We just had so much to chat about, and Tsering Norbu told much a lot of news about mutual acquaintances. Gossiping was a passion that my monk friend shared with the majority of the people of his country.

I longed to start up my beloved "everyday Tibetan life." That meant prostrations at the temple in the morning and visits to Tsering Norbu in the afternoon. He even offered, without my asking, to give me further instruction. Naturally, I had secretly hoped for this. Before I started off on the way home, the monk brought up the topic.

"I will now teach you the high art of breathing. Many

centuries ago, monks developed effective breathing techniques that we practice up to this day. Just like the prostrations, they cleanse the body and mind. These breathing exercises will be good for you."

He didn't want to tell me anymore for the time being. He insisted that I first get some real rest after the strenuous journey.

But there was no recuperation to be had. The landlady at the boardinghouse was namely waiting for me with messages from four Tibetan friends who invited me for the next day. News always spreads like a wildfire in the city, and word of my return had quickly gotten around. I naturally didn't want to decline any of these invitations. So I stood at Tsering Norbu's door the next evening with a belly full of buttered tea and a head full of stories. He just laughed at my latest experience.

"Haven't you learned to maintain a happy medium yet? Buddha taught us to live in balance. We must develop a harmonious equilibrium between taking and giving. Taking in too much is just as intolerable and bad as an excess of giving. Because you had to eat too much, you now have a fully belly and are lazy. The same principle functions for the mind: if you take in too much, you become blocked. You have just experienced all of this."

Tsering Norbu was quite right, but I really didn't have any desire to philosophize at the moment. "Can't we talk about this tomorrow," I asked him feebly, "I'm simply too exhausted."

He hesitated for a moment and at the same time pressed his index finger against the tip of his nose. That was one of his gestures when he was thinking of something special. He took a deep breath and declared in a decisive tone: "Stay here. I will now teach you a very simple and effective breathing technique. You will feel better afterwards. I actually had planned to first tell you a bit about the theory of breathing. But what opportunity will be more favorable for convincing you now, when you need it, of the effectiveness of the exercise? For a change of pace, you will comprehend this by way of practical experience instead of through your intellect."

I admitted defeat. Tsering Norbu directed me to a small rug located in the corner of the room and got a cushion.

"Sit down here. As I said, you have taken in too much information today. This caused a congestion of energy in your body. This exercise will cleanse you. You will visualize colors, which lets you dissolve this congestion and start your natural energy flowing again. Like a pressure-relief valve, you will exhale the excess of information. Now close your eyes, relax, and listen to my voice."

"Imagine the air that you inhale to be completely golden, a golden stream that flows into you from the expanse of the universe. This air is very fresh, light, and made of transparent gold. Let this gold stream into your body. At the same time, calmly and evenly breathe this pure gold into every cell of your body. When you exhale, let a heavy, black stream flow out of your nose. Now associate everything that is heavy and all your thoughts with this stream and let it out. Send this black stream far away, up into the universe. The next time you inhale, once again bring the golden stream into yourself. Completely dissolve your body in this bright light. Every fiber in you becomes relaxed. Your head also becomes very light, flooded with golden light."

I don't know how much time passed. Tsering Norbu had long stopped speaking as I continued to sit on the rug with closed eyes, still flooded with golden light. He let me rest until he thought it was enough. With a pert: "Well, how do you feel now?" my teacher brought me back to reality. He just grinned as I told him in amazement how much clearer my head now was. I actually felt significantly fresher than before.

"Do you know," he ruminated, "rationally-oriented people like you have no difficulty in remembering things. The greater art lies in forgetting what is unimportant. When you exhale the useless chatter, you separate the mental chaff from the wheat. By the way, you can also regulate too much energetic pressure or energy holes in the individual parts of the body with this exercise. Breathe golden light into the respective organ in case of an energy hole. Let the light spread within it and fill the weak area with strength. If you have pain somewhere, imagine it as a mass of black and strongly exhale it."

This first breathing exercise later became a constant companion in my everyday life. It's particularly ideal in the morning after heavy dreams and before going to sleep. A thousand bits of thoughts that have surfaced during the day or night are then exhaled. New space can be created within the mind.

During the day it's also useful to take short breaks while working and inhale the golden light for a moment. The exercise refreshes the concentration for the next activities. There are enough opportunities to do this in hectic everyday life: like when I'm waiting at the supermarket check-out stand or at the post office, when I ride the subway or stand at the bus stop. I now fill such supposedly "empty moments" with conscious breathing, evenly and slowly inhaling the golden light and letting it flow pleasurably through my body. Such moments are invigorating, refreshing, and relaxing! Between all the demands of the day, I could do much good for myself with it.

I later recommended this exercise to a girlfriend who often suffered from headaches. She told me enthusiastically: "Through this conscious way of exhaling, I can already ward off the first hints of a headache. I simply imagine it to be a mass of black and breathe it out. As a result, I permit myself to take a short break at the same time." It had become clear to her that the headaches always occurred when she took on too much. She later made sure that such stress situations didn't even have the chance to arise.

"Your breath is the umbilical cord that connects you with this life," Tsering Norbu lectured some days after my first experience with this wonderful exercise.

"Your life begins with the first and ends with the last breath. But your breath is also a mirror of yourself: It namely reflects precisely the state of your energy. So you know that your breath flows calmly when you are relaxed. As soon as you are nervous or agitated, you breathe in a hectic, choppy way and literally have to gasp for air. This is normal. The breathing functions are namely controlled by the autonomous nervous system. Your body therefore reacts to your emotional state, which is a vital function of nature, by the way.

Imagine that our ancestors were threatened by a wild tiger during the hunt. It is logical that they would no longer breathe in a relaxed manner. To the contrary, their breath would stop short in fright so that they could take to their heels and run away. Nature has then built in the stress factor in a meaningful way. But what you in the West understand as stress has long stopped being healthy. The brief fear of the tiger has become a constant strain: people always say things like 'I have to hurry and go here and there' and 'I have to take care of something.' The nervous system is then permanently overstimulated. It really would be good for you to slow down a bit.

But back to breathing: This connection between the nervous system and breathing fortunately also occurs in the reverse direction: when you regulate your breathing, you influence your nervous system. The breathing exercises have an effective impact at this point. When your breathing is in a state of equilibrium, your soul and your emotions are in balance."

Tsering Norbu looked at me attentively. "Have you understood everything up to now?" I nodded. "Then I have an assignment for you: touch the energy of your breath. Connect your attention with the air you inhale. Each breath will then become an inexhaustible source of invigorating energy. I hope you believe me since your last exercise. Do you know what?" Once again he tapped the tip of his nose with his index finger. "A lesson on breathing is at its loveliest where the air is the best. We are going to take an excursion into the mountains tomorrow!"

That was an outstanding idea. I had seldom experienced my old teacher in such an adventurous mood. When I appeared at his place the next morning with laced hiking boots, he was already prepared. He brought out a backpack filled to bursting with him.

"What do you have in there?" I curiously wanted to know.

"A secret," he smiled. "You will find out soon enough." We climbed into the bus and rode for about an hour, until Tsering Norbu made a sign. "This is where we get out." There was no settlement to be seen anywhere. I secretly asked myself where we were going to get something to eat on the way. While we walked up the path to a delicate green spring meadow, we talked about Buddha and the world.

In the shade of a mighty block of granite, we sat down in satisfaction. We had gotten out of breath, and neither of us spoke a word. This massive mountain range emanated an imperturbable repose and strength. For a moment, the confusing flights of fancy and raging abysses of a human soul dissolve within it.

Tsering Norbu got up and walked to a stream that murmured a few steps from our camp. "Come, you can go ahead and drink the water here. It is very clear and clean." We scooped up some handfuls out of the stream and drank. It tasted wonderful.

"But now to our topic." The old monk was now very serious. "You can put your pad aside. Much of what I will tell you today will seem strange to you. You should therefore concentrate instead on my words so that you understand everything." I leaned back against the granite block and looked at the steel-blue sky in concentration.

"Today is a special day for you. I will initiate you into the breathing exercises. They are the most effective and fascinating breathing exercises that I know. They originate for the most part from an old Buddhist school of the Red Hat Order. For many centuries, monks have practiced these exercises in order to keep their body and mind healthy. Even today, Tibetan doctors prescribe the breathing techniques to their patients in addition to herb pills, diet, and massages.

Take note of the following: Breathing is inseparably connected with the subtle energies that flow through the entire human being. The main energy is connected with the throat center. The flow of energy is created and coordinated for its path through the body in the larynx. This is why the old tradition depicts the throat center as a flower with 16 petals. These petals twine into the various parts of the body. When you breathe evenly and calmly through the mouth and nose, the throat center can develop its full potential. The throat then distributes its energy through these petals into all the regions of the body.

In our Tibetan psychology, the breath has still a further function. According to it, breathing is the foundation of all emotional influences upon the body. Imagine the breath as a horse and the mind as its rider. This 'breath-horse' promotes spiritual qualities and feelings into all of the cells. Now it depends on the type of feelings you have. If you are always unhappy, your body will become ill sooner or later. If you are in a good mood, your breath-horse will feed all the organs with positive information. Your body will become awake and animated, your hearing will become sharpened, and your eyes can more intensively perceive the colors. By breathing attentively, you establish a spiritual relationship to all parts of the body. Connect the breath-horse with all regions of your body, and you will feel yourself more intensively.

These are the most important points that you must know for the time being. Now I will explain the course of the energy channels in the body to you. They are important for the exercises. Imagine the crown chakra, heart chakra, and lower belly to be connected with each other through a thick, straight central channel. Two side channels start at the left and right nostril and lead up to the root of the nose. From there, they run down both sides of the thick central channel back down to the lower belly and flow into it there.

We are now going to take a break and then start with the exercises. Let me give you some good advice on them: "Sink into your body and connect yourself with your breath. You will see that all the sense let you perceive them directly."

Tsering Norbu now got up and stretched his legs a bit. I walked back to the stream. The monk suddenly clapped his hands: "My goodness, I almost forgot something because of all this talk." He got his backpack and unloaded it. Various jars with delicious curry vegetables, some chicken legs, bread, and vegetables appeared. He had lugged this complete meal, including the dishes, all the way up here.

"I made these this morning," he proudly explained and heaped a big spoon of the vegetables on my plate. We enjoyed these delicacies with great relish. During the next hours, Tsering Norbu taught me these special breathing techniques.

It was already late afternoon when we finished our open-air lessons. I had been so busy with the microcosms of my body during the exercises that I had hardly noticed how the sun disappeared behind the mountains. But now I began to freeze and was glad that I had brought along a thick sweater to be on the safe side. Such extreme temperature fluctuations were typical for the climate in Tibet. While the air often shimmered with heat during the day, the thermometer rapidly sank in the evening.

As we arrived at Tsering Norbu's house door after our excursion, he asked me to come in for a brief moment.

"I have another present for you," he promised mysteriously and pulled me into his room. What could it be? He rummaged around extensively in the large chest and then pulled out a scroll.

"Open it," he encouraged me.

I untied the string that was wrapped around the pages and unrolled the paper. I scanned the text with wide eyes. Here were exactly the exercises that I had practiced in the afternoon. Explained very clearly and chronologically, Tsering Norbu had written them down for me in English. The current date stood in the upper right corner of the page.

"An initiation into the high art of breathing should be something festive, shouldn't it?" laughed the old monk. "After all, starting today they will accompany your life. To celebrate this day, I will make us a cup of sweet milk-tea."

While he busied himself at the gas cooker, something else occurred to him: "By the way, you do not need to do these exercises in the order shown here. Simply combine them with each other as you like."

It was already getting dark as I walked back to my boardinghouse with the precious scroll under my arm.

The warm shower felt great that evening. The unusual supply of oxygen during the exercises had invigorated my body. I felt fresher than I had for a long time, as if every cell had been bathed in oxygen. That night I slept as soundly as the marmot we had observed at the stream in the afternoon.

The next morning, I read through the scroll attentively once again:

Introduction

All breathing exercises are done with crossed legs in a comfortable seated position. While doing them, sit either on a cushion on the ground or on a chair with a straight back. The breathing should always be balanced before starting the exercise. This means: slowly and calmly inhale, then hold your breath for two to five seconds. Slowly and calmly exhale, then hold your breath for two to five seconds. The flow of the breath is gentle and even. While inhaling, imagine a golden stream of energy.

While you do this, keep your concentration focused only on the air streaming in and out. Exhale disruptive thoughts in a friendly manner. The exercise lasts 21 breaths. In order to keep the mind alert, attentively count the number of breaths.

Morning Dew

Gentle breathing through the mouth and nose. At first, pay more attention to inhaling. Exhaling should be done as slowly as possible, and the breath should be as delicate as possible. The body should be perceived intensely while the inhalation slows down even more. Arising thoughts and feelings are exhaled in a calm and purposeful manner, in the consciousness that no emotion is permanent. Now pay attention to the exhalation. Once again, the breath remains soft and even. During the slow exhalation, feel the world of your body. Perceive every organ and all your senses. This state of awareness will soon flow through the entire body. Practice this exercise for ten minutes.

Summer Breeze

Gently breathe into all parts of your body. At the same time, establish contact with the individual regions and let them speak. Listen to what they need. For tension and pain, exhale the excess strain. For insufficient functioning, sent bright energy into the respective organ.

Pain should be visualized as a mass of black and immediately exhaled. Send this negative energy out into the universe as far as possible. Weak points in an organ are strengthened and harmonized by consciously breathing golden light into them. This exercise is particularly recommended in order to harmonize the energy within the individual parts of the body.

The following variation is good if you wish to establish contact with your body on a regular basis:

Breathe into all regions, one after the other: First breathe into the toes and feet. The concentration should gradually wander through the organs of the stomach area, the heart, larynx, and the head region up to the forehead. Feel what the organs want to say and send them loving energy.

Autumn Leaves

This exercise is very popular and widespread in Tibet. It is practiced in differing variations. The three most important forms are described in the following.

The best time to do the exercises is in the morning immediately after you get up or in the evening before going to sleep. This breathing technique frees the mind and body from ballast that has accumulated during a night or day. It renews psychological and physical powers.

Variation 1: Birds of Passage

Inhale very deeply and strongly. If possible, the air should touch the tips of the lungs. Belly and chest are entirely full during the inhalation. Place the right index finger against the right side of the nose and press the nostril firmly shut. Then close the mouth and slowly exhale through the left nostril until the very last bit of air has left it. While exhaling, imagine the breath to be a mass of black that streams from the depths of the belly. All mental attitudes related to clinging, wishing, and attachment flow out of the body with it.

For the next breath, hold the left nostril closed with the left index finger. Inhale deeply through the right nostril down to the tip of the belly. Slowly let the air flow out again. Imagine this used breath to be a cloudy, dark-red stream. It is connected with anger, hatred, rage, and aversion.

In the third breath, fresh energy is breathed up through both nostrils, directly into the front of the head. When exhaling, imagine a cloudy gray stream. It is connected with the type of confusion and dullness that is so typical for the human mental condition. Repeat this cycle of three for a total of seven times.

The classic Tibetan tradition associates the following images with this exercise:

Birds stream out of the mass of black from the left nostril. Snakes comes out of the right nostril, and pigs come from the head. These animals symbolize the roots of perpetual human suffering: greed, hatred, and ignorance. These three evils are responsible for human beings remaining imprisoned in the eternal cycle of rebirths.

Variation 2: Wind Gust

This variation basically corresponds with Variation 1. However, here the breath comes into contact with the individual organs in the body.

Close the right nostril and breathe in through the left nostril. The golden, pure stream of air flows down through the neck, chest, navel, and hips to the lower belly. As black energy connected with the feeling of greed, it streams back out of the body. In your thoughts, send this black stream far out into the universe. This possessive energy is connected with the left half of the body. Inhale and exhale three times, whereby the right nostril should always remain closed.

Now hold the left nostril closed. Breathe into the right half of the body through the right nostril: through the throat, heart, navel, and liver down to the gallbladder. Bile represents rage and anger. Breathe these aggressions far out into the universe. Repeat this three times as well.

Now put both hands on your knees in a relaxed position. Breathe up through both nostrils directly into the head three times. The gray breath that pours down connects itself with depression, headaches, circling thoughts, tension, etc.

Variation 3: Blossom Path

The third variation of this breathing technique is connected to a yoga exercise.

Take one deep breath through both nostrils. While doing so, lift both elbows and shoulders and count to five. Then close the right nostril with the right index finger and exhale evenly and gently on the left side. At the same time, count to five and then lower the elbows again. Repeat three times.

Now inhale through both nostrils and simultaneously lift the elbows and shoulders. This time, close the left nostril and breathe out on the right side. Lower the elbows. Also repeat this three times.

Without interrupting, now lift both elbows and breathe through both nostrils. When exhaling, bend the upper body forwards until the head and arms lie on the ground. Count to five while doing this. Now inhale while the head and arms are lifted and sink back to the ground with the following exhalation. Repeat three times.

The effect of this exercise is intensified through the visualization of colors and feelings as described in Variations 1 and 2.

The Rainbow

Tsering Norbu made some notes about these exercises in the margin, which I would like to mention first: "Remember the principle of body, language, and mind," he wrote. "The physical aspect is represented by the head. The language is located in the throat, and the heart symbolizes the mind. Each of these three aspects is connected with a basic syllable. By the way, these basic syllables are older than Buddhism itself. The ancient people of India had already made use of them. These syllables let your body vibrate as soon as you articulate them. They influence the nervous system and thereby have a direct

effect on its centers. The Tibetans know a series of basic syllables. The sounds belonging to this exercise are: OM AH
HUM." So much for his notes.

This was written in the scroll itself about the exercise:

Imagine a figure floating about 30 centimeters in front of
you in free space. This can be the figure of Buddha or any
other being. It is important that it emanates qualities that you
find worthy of striving for. This figure is golden and pervaded
with glittering light. It sits on a golden lotus leaf. The figure
radiates golden light in all directions of the heavens.

First direct your attention to the perfect physical energy
of this deity. White light streams from the top of its head and
floods the entire body. All physical tensions are dissolved in
this white light. Illness and the tendency to treat your body
badly vanish. Now recite the basic syllable OM several times,
and let the OM flow through all your fibers. Your entire body
is pervaded with joy and a feeling of floating. Continue sens-
ing this lightness.

Now direct your attention to this deity's throat center.
It represents released emotional and language-related energy
and streams towards us in a red color. The red light streams
from its throat to our throat and floods it with strength. All
obstacles that stand in the way of the creative expression of
vital energy are dissolved. Blockades that hinder personal development are also dissolved. The red awakens strength, energy, courage, and liveliness. During this visualization, let the
basic syllable AH stream throughout your entire body.

In conclusion, direct your attention to the heart center of
the deity. The heart symbolizes mental energy and radiates as
a blue HUM. The calming, cool blue helps you achieve a clear
view of reality. False hopes and ideas of a so-called reality are
dissolved in this blue. All obstacles that block a clear view of
reality are driven away. The blue color streams cooly through
the body and calms the agitated mind. There is pleasant re-
laxation while the HUM is recited several times.

After reading this, I rolled the texts back up. For me, the visualized figure of the Rainbow Exercise soon became Tara, the feminine goddess for protection and strength. I imagined Tara as a perfect being. She possessed all the qualities that I would also like to have. This type of help was completely legitimate in Tsering Norbu's eyes.

"Whatever figure you most like to visualize," he said, "is a matter of your own personal taste. However, in the course of time you yourself will approach this ideal and become increasingly similar to it the more intensively you dedicate yourself to it."

The Wheel Comes Full Circle

Tsering Norbu was no great friend of ceremony. He therefore had an unperturbed reaction to my impending departure.

"It is good that you have been in Tibet once again," he declared on the day I had to pack my backpack.

"Now you can connect the breathing exercises with the prostrations. Both are perfect techniques that will lend wings to both your everyday life and your spiritual development."

"You could at least be a bit crushed as well," I grumbled, slightly hurt about his indifference. Saying good-bye was difficult enough for me. In these past weeks, Tsering Norbu had become more than my teacher. He had become one of my best friends. Bittersweet melancholy spread in the pit of my stomach. Yet, I knew: he had also blossomed while I was here. And this was not just because of our frequently amusing conversations and some excursions that we'd taken together. This monk was glad that he was allowed to convey his wisdom from a long, fulfilled life to a thankful student.

However, Tsering Norbu didn't want to share that sadness with me.

"Life is like the course of a river," he mused. "Sometimes its water bubbles excitedly through narrow gorges and leaps freshly over stones. Then again, when it flows through broad plains it is like a languid river. What do you think: Can the water stop somewhere? Does it cling to a boulder? No, it naturally doesn't. The river of our lives runs through various levels in the same way. You cannot stop it. Not being too close to the one thing and too far from the other, this is the magic principle. This is why you should see all things to be of equal value, no matter what may come. The river of your life can only flow into the ocean of endless wisdom when it has gathered all the experiences. This is why you should never come to a standstill."

Tsering Norbu looked critically at me. "You see, this is

why I am not sad when you go. Because your river must once again flow to the west. My home, on the other hand, is here in Tibet. You have heard many valuable pieces of wisdom and insights into the nature of the mind. You have experienced initiations into the prostrations and the fulfillment in breathing. This is a great gift. But understand that your happiness is independent of time and space. You can find this happiness just as easily in Europe or somewhere else in the world as you can find it in Tibet.

As long as you encounter your life in openness, nothing and no one can do you harm. Never forget that life should be fun and bring joy. Look at this world as a playground where you collect experiences.

So now go back home in good cheer and with a light heart. And be the architect of your own fortune. Do you remember? Only a satisfied person has a positive effect on his environment."

"You say that my river will flow to the west. But where is your river running?" I asked. The old man now hesitated for a moment. Finally, he questioningly shrugged his shoulders. "I believe my river is running against gravity. It will flow back up the mountain."

I found this answer to be rather absurd. What did Tsering Norbu want to express with it?

Long after I had returned home, this strange sentence occupied my mind. Did he have visions of his approaching death? Although this thought frightened me, I still couldn't believe it somehow because my friend was in the best of health. And his letter also showed no indication of a threatening illness.

One day, a letter from Tsering Norbu once again waited in my mailbox. I opened the wrinkled envelope and scanned the paper while I was still on the stairs. In his familiar handwriting, he had first written about trivial things. Then my eyes were caught by a paragraph. The same sentence that had been on my mind for months was written here once again: "The time has come: my river will now flow uphill against gravity."

I took two steps at once and ran up the last few stairs into the house. There were no details in the letter. He was fine, and I didn't have to worry about him. "I have already sold my house. I can put the money to good use on the mountain. I cannot give you a new postal address. I do not even know exactly where I will live myself. But it will be very remote."

It continued: "I have tried to give you the most important guidelines for a happy life on your path. Now it is up to you to make use of them. As far as I'm concerned, my wheel has come full circle: I will return to my origins."

Since Tsering Norbu, as I have mentioned, was no friend of ceremony, he tersely thanked me for our friendship at the conclusion of his letter. With a simple greeting, he said good-bye. For always, it appeared to me.

Darn, what did all of this mean? My next letters remained unanswered. Was it my concern about his whereabouts or simply a good excuse for the next trip? Perhaps it was also an attack of sentimentality: in any case, I once again had a ticket to Tibet in my pocket the following summer. I wanted, and had to, find my teacher once again. Although Tsering Norbu was of the opinion that I could walk alone—I definitely had the need to return to him.

The people in the city didn't have any exact information about where my teacher was. "I heard that he moved into a cave somewhere," my landlady told me. "But I haven't seen him in months. Just a moment." She wrinkled her forehead and put her index finger on her lower lip. "He's been away since February. I met him at the New Year's festival at the market square. Exactly, that was the last time." I had also received the last letter from him in February.

In the course of the next few days, I scraped together some sparse information about Tsering Norbu. It was astounding that he apparently had had no close friends. No one knew his present

108

whereabouts. He had practically fallen into oblivion. The idea that this trip should be in vain was quite disappointing.

However, one evening someone knocked loudly on the door of my room. Tashi Lhamo stood in the hallway. She was one of the vegetable saleswomen at the market square.

"I have a hot tip for you," she proudly announced. With an expression of importance, the old gossip sat down on the stool that I gave her. She looked at me expectantly.

"Go ahead and tell me," I urged, "but please speak slowly." My Tibetan was fairly good in the meantime, but it didn't tolerate any rhetorical waterfalls.

"A man bought three sacks of white cabbage at my stand today. He muttered something about a hermit for whom he was supposed to bring along a larger supply of vegetables. I naturally started asking questions. The farmer said that this monk lives in a cave quite close to his place. So, what I want to say is: according to the description, it must be Tsering Norbu, although the old man didn't know his name."

"And where does this man live?" My fingers were suddenly as cold as ice. "A two day's journey to the west from here on a secluded farm. I don't know any more details."

My hopes slipped sheerly into the ground. "How should I ever be able to find this place?" I lamented in disappointment.

Tashi Lhamo grinned. "When will you understand: fate is well-disposed towards you since it sent this man to my stand. He will come by my stand tomorrow morning to pick up the sack of potatoes he ordered. Simply wait for him there."

With two mules in tow, the Tibetan actually appeared the next morning.

"I'm already on the way home, he growled and tied down his sacks meticulously on the back mule, "wanted to take along the potatoes as well."

"One moment, please," I now hastily joined in the conversation. "Do you know Tsering Norbu?"

"Who? No, I don't know him."

"I mean the hermit who lives in the cave." This person was extremely sullen. "What does he look like?"

The man described his approximate age and physical stature in a complicated way. There was no doubt—it must be Tsering Norbu.

"May I come with you? Tsering Norbu is my friend, and I must see him."

The Tibetan permitted me to do so. I ran as fast as lightening back to my room and packed the absolute essentials for my trip. This old Tibetan was taciturn like most people who have lived alone too long. We silently walked along the path that clung to the mountain ridge into the horizon. I was quite happy to have this silence because I now had enough time to prepare for the encounter with Tsering Norbu. How should I explain my visit to him? No appropriate sentence occurred to me. So I decided to allow enough space for spontaneity in the coming meeting.

"It's just one more hour from here," the Tibetan interrupted our silence. We had reached his house. He untied the ropes in order to free the animals from their heavy burden.

"Do you want to walk up there tomorrow?" he asked tersely. It was now late afternoon. Against the shimmering sunlight, my glance glided up a narrow side valley located at a slant behind the house. So Tsering Norbu lived somewhere up there.

"No," I responded decisively, "I'm going now."

"Always stay on the path. Then you can see the cave to the left halfway up the cliff. You can't miss it at all. And tell him that I'll bring up his barley and vegetables with the mules tomorrow," he called behind me. I had almost reached the next bend.

It was dry up here. Barren and lonely. How would the winter be? Thoughts shoot through my mind, coming and flattering away again with the icy wind. On the stony, narrow path, I startle two or three rock goats. They flee in fright, surprised to see a human being.

Now I am standing in front of the cave. No sound. Just

my heart throbbing in my throat up to the roots of my hair. A wooden board leans in front of the entrance to the cave, probably meant to be a door. I hesitantly approach it and knock softly against the wood. The sound echoes from the mountains across the valley and causes me to flinch. Or was it just a gust of wind that grabs the collar of my parka at this moment and whistles sharply into its neckline?

Paper rustles inside the door, and then there are shuffling steps. The heavy wooden board is slowly hoisted to the side. A body becomes visible as a silhouette against the dark cave hole. We stand silently facing each other for a moment. Only then do I see Tsering Norbu's familiar, arch grin: "Snowy air today. Do you feel the wind?"

He takes a step to the side and lets me enter. The next moment, I hear him rustling in the corner. As far as I can tell, he is putting on the water. Everything is almost like before. I'm happy that I don't have to say anything now.

A little while later, my eyes perceive silhouettes in the unaccustomed darkness. Two mattresses, a wooden table, and a gigantic metal box, which I already know from his old apartment. It serves as both a closet for his clothes and storage space for his papers. In the corner there is an altar with some bronze Buddha statues and all kinds of treasures on it. The burning butter lamp flickers as I walk to the altar. All of these objects are familiar to me and make the room surprisingly cozy. I prefer to push aside thoughts about the approaching bitterly cold winter.

"You are truly a determined student," I now hear his teasing voice behind me. "You visit me at this end of the world! The tea still needs a moment." We sit across from each other on the two mattresses. Tsering Norbu asks whether I had a good journey and wants to know how life is treating me. While we chat, the old familiarity weaves its fine threads between our souls. Everything is like it was before—but just almost because my friend and teacher has changed since our last encounter.

His face has become thinner, or rather, more ascetic. His dark eyes sparkle in a way that is lively and oddly distant at the same time, like stars that are light years away. The red monk's robe hangs loose from his body, yet he moves just as supple as before. Never before have I experienced such a concurrence of presence and the certainty that this spirit floats in completely different spheres at the same time.

This change in my friend both fascinates and frightens me. Some time passes before I summon up the courage to ask my burning question. At some point I hear my own voice echo from the dark stone walls: "Why are you here? Why did you say back then that your stream is running uphill?"

Startled by my own loudness, I recoil. Tsering Norbu smiles at me calmly, and his dark eyes even become a bit blacker. Warm love and endless clarity comes from the depths of these eyes, reaching directly into my heart. Later, whenever I call this memory to mind, an affectionate shiver floods through me: Tsering Norbu was connected with the most profound perception of all-embracing wisdom at this moment. This is why I now already know the answer before he opens his mouth:

"Do you still remember that many yogis retreat into the solitude of meditation for three years and three months? It is also time for me to harvest the fruits of my life. The wheel of human existence therefore comes full circle. You come from the silence, and one day you return to the silence. I am now preparing myself for this. My spiritual practice helps me calm my inner nature. Do you see," he indicates the valley outside with an inclusive sweep of the arm, "there is no distraction here, no noise, no people. I love this stillness."

With a deep sigh of satisfaction, Tsering Norbu now looks at me. I bite on my lower lip in uncertainty.

"Then you will be back in the city in about three years."

"Now just stop that nonsense," the old monk reprimands

me in a fatherly way. "Haven't you learned yet to have a minimum of openness and imperturbability?" While he says this, he puts his bony hand on my arm in a reconciliatory manner.

"Simply have trust in life. Most things take care of themselves. It doesn't matter whether you plan them or not. Listen to your inner voice in unshakeable trust and let yourself be guided by it. How should I know where my future is leading me."

The silence stands like an impenetrable wall between us for a while. We suddenly have no more topics to discuss. Yet, as always, Tsering Norbu is more composed than I am.

"Do you notice anything special in my new palace," he asks almost coquettishly. Irritated, I let my eyes wander around the room and notice one little thing or another. He always shakes his head.

"What is it that I should notice?"

With a grin, he points at a slant behind himself. "Look. I have let enough room for my prostrations here. I practice them every day for half-an-hour. At least."

Now I smile more freely. "Prostrations are the essence of all yogas in a bud, aren't they?"

"Clever student. Even we great yogis practice the prostrations up to the point of our enlightenment."

Relieved, I join him as he laughs. At this moment, the wheel of our friendship also comes full circle. Satisfied and with a wistful ache in the chest, I slip back into my jacket. Will this good-bye be forever? But Tsering Norbu doesn't leave me any time for melancholy thoughts. A friendly hug, as unspectacular as always, and then he calls after me as I walk down the path: "And tell the farmer that he should definitely bring up the vegetables tomorrow."

"I'll see to it, you can depend on me," I call up to his cave against the icy wind.

I walk down the narrow ravine in a trance. The encounter of this past hour once again runs through my head like an unreal film. Even if this world isn't my world—I can still take a part of it with me.

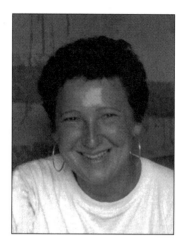

The Author

Jutta Mattausch, born in 1961, is a successful journalist who works for prominent magazines and newspapers. She has traveled to almost all Asian countries and acquired deep knowledge of the Tibetan culture.

In 1994, she established a school in a Himalayan village, which allows all children, irrespective of their financial possibilities, to receive a good education and become acquainted with their cultural traditions.

If you would like to write Jutta Mattausch or tell her about your own experiences with the practice of the "Tibetan Power Yoga," then write her with a self-addressed, stamped return envelope in care of the Windpferd Verlag. We will give the letter to the author.

Windpferd Verlag
"Tibetan Power Yoga"
Postfach
87648 Aitrang, Germany

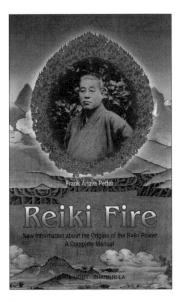

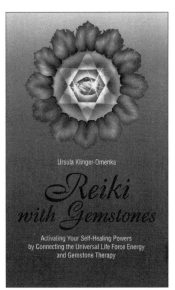

Frank Arjava Petter

Reiki Fire

New Information about the Origins of the Reiki Power
A Complete Manual

The origin of Reiki has come to be surrounded by many stories and myths. The author, a free Reiki master practicing in Japan, immerses it in a new light as he traces Usui-san's path back through time with openness and devotion. He meets Usui's descendants and climbs the holy mountain of his enlightenment. Reiki, shaped by Shintoism, is a Buddhist expression of Qigong, whereby Qigong depicts the teaching of life energy in its original sense. An excellent textbook, fresh and rousing in its spiritual perspective and an absolutely practical Reiki guide. The heart, the body, the mind, and the esoteric background, it is all here.

144 pages, $12.95
ISBN 0-914955-50-0

Ursula Klinger-Omenka

Reiki with Gemstones

Activating Your Self-Healing Powers —Connecting the Universal Life Force Energy with Gemstone Therapy

While Reiki, the universal life energy, brings the physical and emotional functions back into their original harmony, gemstones concentrate light-filled powers and color vibrations into the chakras, whose unrestricted functioning is greatly important for vitality and well-being. By connecting Reiki with gemstone therapy, the powers of self-healing are activated in a natural manner. The author writes on the basis of many years of rich experience in working with Reiki and gemstones. She trustingly places her perceptions into the hands of the reader, who can put them to practical use for the good of all beings within a short time.

128 pages, $12.95
ISBN 0-914955-29-2

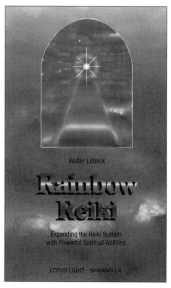

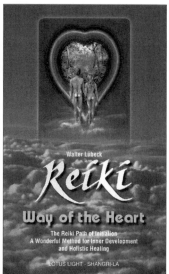

Walter Lübeck

Rainbow Reiki

Expanding the Reiki System with Powerful Spiritual Abilities

Rainbow Reiki gives us a wealth of possibilities to achieve completely new and different things with Reiki than taught in the traditional system. Walter Lübeck has tested these new methods in practical application for years and teaches them in his courses.

Making Reiki Essences, performing guided aura and chakra work, connecting with existing power places and creating new personal ones, as well as developing Reiki Mandalas, are all a part of this system. This work is accompanied by plants devas, crystal teachers, angels of healing stones, and other beings of the spiritual world.

192 pages, $14.95
ISBN 0-914955-28-4

Walter Lübeck

Reiki—Way of the Heart

The Reiki Path of Initiation
A Wonderful Method for Inner Development and Holistic Healing

Reiki—Way of the Heart is for everyone interested in the opportunities and experiences offered by this very popular esoteric path of perception, based on easily learned exercises conveyed by a Reiki Master to students in three degrees.

If you practice Reiki, the use of universal life energy to heal oneself and others, you will have the possibility of receiving direct knowledge about your personal development, health, and transformation.

Walter Lübeck also presents a good survey of various Reiki schools and shows how Reiki can be applied successfully in many areas of life.

192 pages, $ 14.95
ISBN 0-941524-91-4

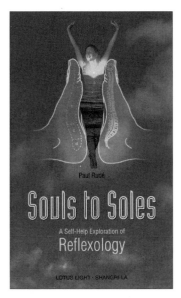

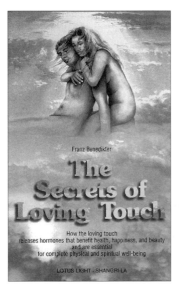

Paul Rudé

Souls to Soles

A Self-Help Exploration of Reflexology

Caring for the feet has been part of the culture of many civilizations, for thousands of years. Now bursting forth all over the world, reflexology is being widely accepted as a safe, powerful means of reducing stresses, promoting vitality and well-being. The author has masterfully captured the essence of reflexology with beautiful illustrations and clearly presented guides for using your touch effectively on the feet. Truly an exploration, this book takes you on a fun loving adventure that has value for all age groups. Breaking new ground, this book also shows you how to reach out to the young, to help them in their times of discomfort, a tender loving experience for those who cannot help themselves.

160 pages, $12.95
ISBN 0-914955-51-9

Franz Benedikter

The Secrets of Loving Touch

How the Loving Touch Releases Hormones that Benefit Health, Happiness, and Beauty and Are Essential for Complete Physical and Spiritual Well-Being

Psychologist Franz Benedikter helps readers create the best possible hormonal basis for a healthy, happy, and liberated life. A release of relaxing, activating, and euphoretic hormones occurs when certain trigger zones of the body are gently touched. With this compact exercise program, we can have a positive effect on the body, mind, and soul through a form of self-massage and partner massage that is more like a loving touch. Since every healthy person has a longing to be touched, this book introduces a new age of tenderness.

144 pages, 12.95 $
ISBN 0-941524-90-6

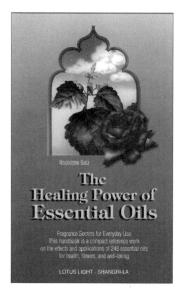

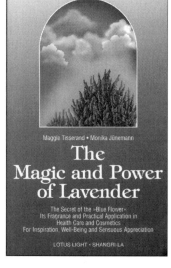

Rodolphe Balz

The Healing Power of Essential Oils

Fragrance Secrets for Everyday Use. This handbook is a compact reference work on the effects and applications of 248 essential oils for health, fitness, and well-being

Fifteen years of organic cultivation of spice plants and healing herbs in the French Provence have provided Rodolphe Balz with extensive knowledge about essential oils, how they work, and how to use them.

The heart of *The Healing Power of Essential Oils* is an essenial-oil index describing their properties, followed by a comprehensive therapeutic index for putting them to practical use. Further topics of this indispensible aromatherapy handbook are distillation processes, concentrations, chemotypes, quality and quality control, toxicity, self-medication, and the aromatogram.

208 pages, $ 14.95
ISBN 0-941524-89-2

Magie Tisserand · Monika Jünemann

The Magic and Power of Lavender

The Secret of the Blue Flower

The scent of lavender practically has permeated whole regions of Europe, contributing to their special character, and dominated perfumery for most of its history. To this very day, lavender has remained one of the most familiar, popular, and utilized of all fragrances.

This book introduces you to the delightful and enticing secrets of this plant and its essence, demonstrating its healing power, while also presenting the places and people involved in its cultivation. The authors have asked doctors, holistic health practitioners, chemists, and perfumers about their experiences and share them – together with their own with you.

136 pages, $ 9.95
ISBN 0-941524-88-4

AYURVEDA AND PANCHAKARMA
The Science of Healing and Rejuvenation

SUNIL V. JOSHI M.D. (AYU)

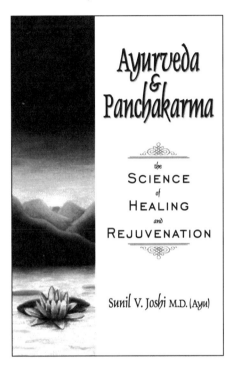

"The treasurehouse of Ayurvedic wisdom is accessible to more people through this wonderful book of Dr. Sunil Joshi. His knowledge and experience in Ayurvedic purification (Panchakarma) has been invaluable to our programs at The Chopra Center for Well Being."

DEEPAK CHOPRA M.D.
AUTHOR, *Ageless Body, Timeless Mind*

PUBLISHED BY LOTUS PRESS
To order your copy, send $19.95 plus $3.00 postage and handling ($1.50 each add'l copy) to:

Lotus Press
P O Box 325TPY
Twin Lakes, Wi 53181 USA
Request our complete book and alternative health products catalogs of over 7000 items. Wholesale inquiries welcome.

Sources of Supply:

The following companies have an extensive selection of useful products and a long track-record of fulfillment. They have natural body care, aromatherapy, flower essences, crystals and tumbled stones, homeopathy, herbal products, vitamins and supplements, videos, books, audio tapes, candles, incense and bulk herbs, teas, massage tools and products and numerous alternative health items across a wide range of categories.

WHOLESALE:

Wholesale suppliers sell to stores and practitioners, not to individual consumers buying for their own personal use. Individual consumers should contact the RETAIL supplier listed below. Wholesale accounts should contact with business name, resale number or practitioner license in order to obtain a wholesale catalog and set up an account.

Lotus Light Enterprises, Inc.

P O Box 1008 TPY
Silver Lake, WI 53170 USA
414 889 8501 (phone)
414 889 8591 (fax)
800 548 3824 (toll free order line)

RETAIL:

Retail suppliers provide products by mail order direct to consumers for their personal use. Stores or practitioners should contact the wholesale supplier listed above.

Internatural

33719 116th Street TPY
Twin Lakes, WI 53181 USA
800 643 4221 (toll free order line)
414 889 8581 office phone
WEB SITE: www.internatural.com

Web site includes an extensive annotated catalog of more than 7000 products that can be ordered "on line" for your convenience 24 hours a day, 7 days a week.